Physical Therapy Documentation

▶ From Examination to Outcome

THIRD EDITION

Physical Therapy Documentation

From Examination to Outcome

THIRD EDITION

Mia L. Erickson, PT, EdD
Certified Hand Therapist
Physical Therapy Department
Midwestern University
Glendale, Arizona

Ralph R. Utzman, PT, MPH, PhD
Professor and Director of Clinical Education
Division of Physical Therapy
West Virginia University School of Medicine
Morgantown, West Virginia

Rebecca S. McKnight, PT, MS
Educational Consultant
Reach Consulting, LLC
Forsyth, Missouri

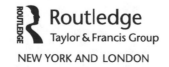

Routledge
Taylor & Francis Group

NEW YORK AND LONDON

Physical Therapy Documentation: From Examination to Outcome, Third Edition includes ancillary materials specifically available for faculty use, including PowerPoint Slides. Please visit www.routledge.com/9781630916268 to obtain access.

First published 2020 by SLACK Incorporated

Published 2024 by Routledge
605 Third Avenue, New York, NY 10158

and by Routledge
4 Park Square, Milton Park, Abingdon, Oxon OX14 4RN

Routledge is an imprint of the Taylor & Francis Group, an informa business

Library of Congress Cataloging-in-Publication Data
Names: Erickson, Mia L., author. | Utzman, Ralph, 1966- author. | McKnight,
    Rebecca, 1969- author.
Title: Physical therapy documentation : from examination to outcome / Mia
    L. Erickson, Ralph R. Utzman, Rebecca S. McKnight.
Description: Third edition. | Thorofare, NJ : SLACK Incorporated, [2020] |
    Includes bibliographical references and index.
Identifiers: LCCN 2020006208 | ISBN 9781630916268 (paperback) | ISBN
Subjects: MESH: Physical Therapy Specialty--organization & administration |
    Medical Records | Forms and Records Control
Classification: LCC RM725 | NLM WB 460 | DDC 615.8/2--dc23
LC record available at https://lccn.loc.gov/2020006208

Cover Artist: Katherine Christie

ISBN: 9781630916268 (pbk)
ISBN: 9781003525714 (ebk)

DOI: 10.4324/9781003525714

Contents

Acknowledgments

I would like to say thank you to Ralph and Becky for continuing to see the need for this text and for supporting this project. Thank you also for your countless hours of work and contributions. I am also grateful to all the students who have used this text and allowed me to see areas where we needed to improve. This has kept me accountable for providing a high-quality product and striving to make it the best textbook for documentation available. To my family, thank you for allowing me the hours to make this happen.

—*Mia L. Erickson, PT, EdD*

Thank you to Mia Erickson and Becky McKnight for asking me to join them in writing the first edition all those years ago. My participation in this project has strengthened my teaching and clinical documentation skills. I also thank my colleagues and students who have provided helpful feedback and suggestions for the new edition. Finally, thank you to my family and co-workers for their support.

—*Ralph R. Utzman, PT, MPH, PhD*

It has indeed been an honor to continue working with Mia and Ralph on this project. I thank them both for the opportunity. There never is a good time to squeeze in the work necessary to write or revise a textbook, and I appreciate your willingness to shoulder the extra burden and keep this resource available to physical therapy programs and students.

I also want to thank my husband and my daughter for putting up with me when I cloister myself to work on projects like this. Thank you for your patience, your support, and your unconditional love.

—*Rebecca S. McKnight, PT, MS*

About the Authors

Mia L. Erickson, PT, EdD is Professor and Assistant Program Director at Midwestern University in Glendale, AZ. Mia holds a bachelor's degree from West Virginia University in Secondary Education and a Master of Science degree in Physical Therapy from the University of Indianapolis. She earned her Doctor of Education degree with emphasis in Curriculum and Instruction from West Virginia University. Her clinical practice is in the area of hand and upper extremity rehabilitation.

Ralph R. Utzman, PT, MPH, PhD is Professor and Director of Clinical Education in the Division of Physical Therapy at the West Virginia University School of Medicine. He earned his bachelor's degree in Physical Therapy and Master of Public Health degree from West Virginia University, and his PhD in Health-Related Sciences from the Medical College of Virginia campus of Virginia Commonwealth University. His clinical practice focuses on patients with balance impairments related to vestibular and neurologic movement disorders. He teaches courses in professional development, health policy, and practice administration. He is a trainer for the American Physical Therapy Association Credentialed Clinical Instructor Program, Levels 1 and 2.

Rebecca S. McKnight, PT, MS received her Bachelor of Science degree in Physical Therapy from St. Louis University in 1992 and her post-professional Master of Science degree from Rocky Mountain University of Health Professions in 1999. Rebecca taught in the Physical Therapist Assistant Program at Ozarks Technical Community College (OTC) in Springfield, MO, from 1997 to 2011, nine of those years serving as Program Director. Currently, Rebecca provides consultation to institutions of higher education related to curriculum and instructional design and student and program-level assessment through her company Reach Consulting. She also is an adjunct Anatomy instructor for OTC.

Preface

Thank you for choosing the third edition of *Physical Therapy Documentation: From Examination to Outcome*. We are excited to provide you with an up-to-date tool for learning the basics of clinical documentation in physical therapy. This book serves mainly as a primer for learning to navigate the medical record and to construct relevant documentation necessary for survival in the current health care environment. It is laid out to present the basics of documentation, such as various formats, rules for writing in medical records, and reasons for documenting. However, the difference between this text and others is that the mechanics of writing are taught in such a way that basic documentation elements are blended with contemporary concepts.

Similar to prior editions, the International Classification of Functioning, Disability and Health disablement framework is used to emphasize the integration of function, results of physical therapy interventions, and patient improvement. We have also continued to emphasize showing the unique skills we provide patients and describing why interventions are medically necessary.

While we introduce the components of SOAP and the components for each section, we are using a more contemporary format in this edition. We hope that readers are provided with information on overall note structure and can adapt into either paper or electronic records. We have also emphasized the need for high-quality content within each section.

We have continued to integrate concepts of evidence-based practice into documentation. More experienced clinicians will also benefit from the information to improving documentation quality in the areas of skilled care and medical necessity. In addition, we provide the reader with examples and practice problems ranging from simple to complex. These examples and problems come from various practice settings and allow the user to develop basic skills and then transition to developing a plan of care, developing progress reports, and writing discharge documentation.

We are happy to provide this to our audience and students of documentation who will carry these concepts into clinical practice. Enjoy.

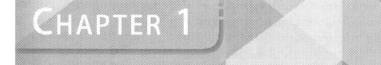

Disablement and Documentation

Mia L. Erickson, PT, EdD

CHAPTER OUTLINE

- Overview of Disablement
- Disablement and Physical Therapy
- Disablement and Documentation

CHAPTER OBJECTIVES

Upon completion of this chapter, the reader will be able to:

1. Define disablement
2. Discuss the need for standard disablement concepts in patient care, health policy, and research
3. Describe the ICF
4. Differentiate between body functions/structures, activities and participation, and contextual factors
5. Differentiate between positive factors and negative contextual factors
6. Describe the components and purpose of the WHO-FIC
7. Examine the integration of disablement in physical therapy practice
8. List ways to integrate disablement concepts into documentation

Erickson ML, Utzman RR, McKnight RS.
*Physical Therapy Documentation: From Examination to Outcome,
Third Edition* (pp 1-6).
© 2020 Taylor & Francis Group.

KEY TERMS

activity
activity limitation
contextual factors
core set
disability
disablement framework
environmental factors
impairment
participation
participation restriction
personal factor

KEY ABBREVIATIONS

ICF
WHO
WHO-FIC

OVERVIEW OF DISABLEMENT

The traditional approach to defining a person's state of health comes from the biomedical model where health means free of, or absent from, disease.[1] The focus of this model is on the biological cause of the disease, illness, or injury, and treatment is aimed at a cure. In the biomedical model, there is often little emphasis on how the disease affects the individual's ability to function or participate in society. A person's health, or state of health, is individualized and is influenced by numerous internal and external factors. A more contemporary meaning of health goes beyond the mere presence or absence of disease, illness, or injury. The World Health Organization (WHO) defined health as a state in which there is complete physical, mental, and social well-being and not merely the absence of disease or infirmity.[2] This approach to health encompasses the biopsychosocial model, an alternative to the biomedical model.[3]

As a health care provider, it is important to recognize the presence of a disease, injury, or illness does not directly correlate with the inability to perform self-care skills, function in the home environment, attain gainful employment, or participate in community or social activities. For example, the same medical diagnosis can impact different people in different ways. Because of the individual nature of health, it is important for health care providers to consider the consequence(s) of any disease, injury, or illness for every patient encountered. Advances in medical care are prolonging the lives of individuals who once may not have survived a chronic disease or severe injury. Yet, increased survival does not equate to restoration of function, social roles, or

quality of life, and individuals surviving life-threatening illnesses can have long-term functional loss, disability, and dependence. These consequences can dramatically influence an individual's ability to function in society and his or her overall quality of life.

The consequences of disease have become known as *disablement*.[4] Disablement frameworks have been developed to categorize or "organize information about the consequences of disease."[5(p5)] The International Classification of Functioning, Disability and Health (ICF) is an example of a disablement framework that was endorsed by the 54th World Health Assembly and released in 2001.[6] It is based on the biopsychosocial model blending anatomical and physiological impairments, physical functioning (including tasks and social roles), and contextual factors (individual and external factors), thus allowing providers to explore different components of a person's health.[7] It provides a common language for health care providers to describe function and dysfunction according to health and health-related states.

The operational definitions listed here have been endorsed by WHO as part of the ICF[6(pp3,12-14)]:

Activity	Completion of a task or action by an individual
Participation	Involvement in a life situation
Functioning	Encompasses bodily functions, activities, and participation
Impairment	A problem with body function (physiological or psychological) or a structure (limb or organ) such as a deviation from or loss of what would be considered normal; impairments may be directly related to the health condition or a result of another impairment (eg, postural abnormalities due to muscle imbalance).
	Impairments can be considered permanent or temporary; progressive, regressive, or static; intermittent or continuous; slight or severe; or fluctuating.
Activity limitations	Difficulties that might be encountered by an individual who is attempting to complete a task or carry out an activity
Participation restrictions	Problems an individual might face while involved in a life situation(s)
Disability	Encompasses impairments, activity limitations, and participation restrictions (Example 1-1)

	PART 1: FUNCTIONING AND DISABILITY		**PART 2:** CONTEXTUAL FACTORS	
COMPONENTS	Body functions and structures	Activities and participation	Environmental factors	Personal factors
DOMAINS	Body functions Body structures	Life areas (tasks, actions)	External influences on functioning and disability	Internal influences on functioning and disability
CONSTRUCTS	Change in body functions (physiological) Change in body structures (anatomical)	Capacity—Executing tasks in a standard environment Performance—Executing tasks in the current environment	Facilitating or hindering impact of features (attributes) of the physical, social, and attitudinal world	Impact of attributes of the person
POSITIVE ASPECT	Functional and structural integrity	Activities Participation	Facilitators	Not applicable
	Functioning			
NEGATIVE ASPECT	Impairment	Activity limitation Participation restriction	Barriers/hindrances	Not applicable
	Disability			

Reprinted with permission from the World Health Organization.

TABLE 1-1

THE INTERNATIONAL CLASSIFICATION OF FUNCTIONING, DISABILITY AND HEALTH FROM THE WORLD HEALTH ORGANIZATION

The ICF categorizes information about an individual's health condition into 2 distinct but related parts: (1) Functioning and Disability and (2) Contextual Factors.[6] Part 1, Functioning and Disability, is further divided into 2 components: (1) Body Functions and Structures and (2) Activities and Participation. Part 2, Contextual Factors, is composed of (1) Environmental Factors and (2) Personal Factors (Table 1-1).

The Body Functions and Structures component of the ICF framework deals with basic anatomical structures and physiological functioning. Under this component, the provider identifies functional and structural integrity and deviations from normal, or impairments. Body structures and systems that are intact are considered positive aspects of health, whereas identified impairments are considered negative aspects of health. Under the Activities and Participation component, activities are defined as "the execution of a task or action."[6(p10)] These are isolated tasks or functional activities such as brushing teeth, combing hair, and dressing. Participation is defined as "involvement in life situations."[8(p4)] Participation includes the performance of socially constructed activities such as work, school, or community involvement. In using the ICF, the examiner

---

Example 1-1. Effects of Disease on Function— Cerebrovascular Accident

Think about the following 2 patients who have had a cerebrovascular accident. Patient A had a small middle carotid artery bleed with little motor and sensory loss. One year later, he is able to safely perform all mobility activities, (eg, walking around the house and the community), self- and home-care activities, and some higher-level thinking activities allowing him to work a part-time job. Patient B, with the same diagnosis of a cerebrovascular accident, had a massive bleed and did not have rapid access to adequate medical care. His clinical presentation was more complex, and the outcome was much less favorable. This patient requires 24-hour care, assistance to move in and out of bed, and a wheelchair for all mobility.

identifies tasks and life situations in which the individual can perform (positive aspects) as well as those in which the individual cannot perform (negative aspects). The online version of the ICF can be found at http://apps.who.int/classifications/icfbrowser/.

According to the WHO,[6] there can be difficulty differentiating between activities and participation. In looking back to the proposed definitions, an *activity* is simply a task or action carried out by an individual, whereas *participation* is involvement in a life situation. The WHO has suggested ways that health care practitioners can operationally define or differentiate between activities and participation within a given setting. These include the following: (1) to designate some functional skills as activities and some as participation (no overlap); (2) to designate some functional skills as activities and some as participation (with overlap); (3) to name detailed skills as activities and broad skills as participation; or (4) to call all skills "activities and participation," not differentiating between the 2.[6]

Contextual factors include environmental and personal factors that influence societal participation, either positively or negatively. Environmental factors are external factors, either immediate or global, that affect the individual as he or she interacts with society. More specifically, they "make up the physical, social and attitudinal environment in which people live and conduct their lives."[6(p16)] Things that facilitate interaction with the environment (ie, wheelchair ramps) are considered *positive aspects*, whereas things that hinder interaction or prevent the individual from participating in the environment are known as *negative aspects*. Examples include others' opinions or attitudes as well as physical barriers such as curbs and stairs. Personal factors are factors that are unique to the individual, such as age, comorbidities, or fitness level. Body Functions, Body Structures, Activities and Participation, and Contextual Factors included within the ICF can be found at http://apps.who.int/classifications/icfbrowser/.

The ICF is one classification system under the World Health Organization Family of International Classifications (WHO-FIC).[7] The primary purpose of the WHO-FIC is to provide a uniform, standard language to describe health, disease, function, disability, and interventions. Other WHO-FIC classification systems are the *International Classification of Diseases, Tenth Revision*, which is a classification system for medical diagnoses and diseases, and the International Classification of Health Interventions, a classification of curative and preventive health interventions currently being beta tested.[9] The 3 classifications are designed to complement one another. Standard classification systems and language facilitate the collection, retrieval, and comparison of disease-related data, which can be useful in clinical settings, research, and policy development.

DISABLEMENT AND PHYSICAL THERAPY

Disablement models have been a topic in physical therapy literature for the last 2 to 3 decades. In 2006, Jette[10] identified a need for a common language in physical therapy clinical practice and research. In this article, several disablement frameworks were discussed, and the author concluded that the ICF held great promise to "provide the rehabilitation disciplines with a universal language with which to discuss disability."[10(p733)] In 2008, the American Physical Therapy Association House of Delegates voted to endorse the ICF, which includes using the ICF language in all future publications, documents, and communications.[11]

Since then, there has been an increase in ICF integration in physical therapy core documents and publications, and it is becoming more prevalent in education, research, and clinical practice.[12] Following a scoping narrative review regarding the use of the ICF in physical therapy, authors found it was being used as a common language for physical therapy practice; as a framework for clinical documentation; and as an aid in developing clinical reasoning, planning care, and establishing treatment goals.[12] The ICF has also been used as a framework for evaluating patient outcome measures and developing clinical practice guidelines and core sets. Core sets facilitate the description of functioning, including body structures and functions, activities and participation, and contextual factors that are essential and relevant for describing specific health conditions.[13] The ICF Research Branch and WHO have developed a rigorous scientific process on developing core sets.[12]

The ICF can be used as a framework for the physical therapy episode of care, especially during the initial examination. During the examination, the physical therapist assesses the patient's body structures and function including his or her ability to complete specific activities and participate in social roles. This allows the physical therapist to identify the positive and negative aspects of the individual's health. Deviations from normal body structure and function are considered impairments. The inability to perform specific activities would be considered activity limitations, whereas the inability to participate in desired life roles would be considered participation restrictions. During the examination, the physical therapist will have to identify contextual factors that facilitate or hinder patient functioning. Using clinical decision making, the physical therapist examines all of the examination data and determines the appropriate intervention strategies necessary to minimize impairments, activity limitations, or participation restrictions.

TABLE 1-2
INTEGRATING DISABLEMENT INTO PHYSICAL THERAPY DOCUMENTATION
Document results of tests and measures that identify or quantify impairments in body structure/function, activity limitations, and participation restrictions.
Documentation describes HOW the impairment(s) are contributing to the activity limitation(s) and participation restriction(s).
Documentation describes HOW the interventions are bringing about change(s) in impairments in body structure/function, activity limitations, and participation restrictions.

DISABLEMENT AND DOCUMENTATION

Documentation, otherwise known as *medical record keeping*, has been defined as "any entry into the individual's health record, such as consultation reports, initial examination reports, progress notes, flow sheets, checklists, re-examination reports, or summations of care—that identifies the care or service provided and the individual's response to intervention."[14] Complete documentation also includes the physician prescription(s) and certification(s), communication with other care providers, copies of exercise programs or patient instructions, as well as any other care providers' notes or comments that support the interventions provided.[15]

There is a need in physical therapy for a common language, or consistency in terminology. One way to accomplish this is through consistency in our documentation, because our "notes" are the sole record of the episode of care provided to each patient or client. Disablement frameworks provide terms and concepts that can be integrated into our documentation to improve consistency in the language used.

Disablement concepts can be integrated and documented throughout the episode of care (Table 1-2). The physical therapy examination will detect the individual's impairments in body structure and function. These are often limitations in range of motion, strength, balance, etc; however, the examination must go beyond the impairment level to identify the consequences of disease and appreciate how the patient's ability to function has been compromised. This includes documenting the patient's ability and inability to perform meaningful activities or tasks, such as hygiene or dressing, and participate in normal life situations, such as work- or school-related functions. It is also important for the physical therapist to describe how the impairment(s) are impacting or causing the functional deficit(s) and vice versa. It is important that function and notations describing the relationship(s) between impairment and function are included so the reader gets a broad view of how the disease, injury, or illness has impacted the patient's overall roles and quality of life.

The physical therapist establishes the prognosis and intervention plan in a manner that addresses the documented impairments, activity limitations, participation restrictions, and contextual factors. Throughout the episode of care, changes in impairment and function brought on by the intervention should be documented and described.

SUMMARY

Disablement, or the consequences of disease, is an important aspect of rehabilitation. Physical therapists need consistency across the profession and a consistent way to communicate with various health care providers. One way to achieve that goal is to integrate disablement terms and concepts. The ICF serves as a framework for the physical therapy episode of care and can be reflected in documentation. The ICF serves as a framework for documentation in this text. As you will read in subsequent chapters, documentation serves many purposes and can be written in a variety of formats; regardless of the style that you are using, your documentation should use consistent disablement terminology.

REVIEW QUESTIONS

1. In your own words, describe disablement.
2. How is the biomedical model different from the biopsychosocial model of health care?
3. List reasons for the need for a disablement framework in physical therapy.

4. What is the difference between a body structure and function?

5. What is the difference between
   a. Activity and participation?
   b. Activity limitations and participation restrictions?

6. What is the difference between an environmental factor and a personal factor? How do they influence an individual's health?

7. What is the difference between a positive factor of health and a negative factor of health?

8. What is the WHO-FIC?

9. What is a core set?

10. How should disablement be reflected in a physical therapist's examination and in documentation?

APPLICATION EXERCISES

For 1 through 10, indicate whether the following is (are) pathology (P), impairment in body structure or function (I), activity limitation (AL), or participation restriction (PR) according to the ICF.

1. Elbow flexion contracture

2. Right hip osteoarthritis

3. A 48-year-old man requires a wheelchair for community mobility and can self-propel 200 feet on level surfaces prior to fatigue

4. Difficulty opening a heavy door

5. A 57-year-old man with impaired mobility is unable to go to the grocery store independently

6. Decreased shoulder range of motion

7. Emphysema

8. Congenital hip dysplasia

9. A 55-year-old man is unable to open a jar because of weakness following a cerebrovascular accident

10. A 15-year-old girl with spastic quadriplegia is unable to participate in physical education class with her peers

For 11 to 15, read the scenario and based on the pathology, list the impairments, activity limitations, and participation restrictions you would expect.

11. A 45-year-old man who has osteoarthritis in the right knee

12. A 76-year-old woman 4 weeks after a left cerebrovascular accident with right hemiplegia

13. A 55-year-old man 4 days after myocardial infarction with a history of type 2 diabetes and high cholesterol

14. A 64-year-old woman with a 3-year history of low back pain

15. A 55-year-old man who underwent a right transtibial amputation 3 weeks ago

REFERENCES

1. MacDermid JC, Law M, Michlovitz SL. Outcome measurement in evidence-based rehabilitation. In: Law M, MacDermid JC, eds. *Evidence-Based Rehabilitation: A Guide to Practice*. Thorofare, NJ: SLACK Incorporated; 2014:65-104.

2. World Health Organization. Constitution of the World Health Organization: principles. https://www.who.int/about/mission/en/. Published 1946. Accessed December 7, 2018.

3. Wade DT, Halligan PW. The biopsychosocial model of illness: a model whose time has come. *Clin Rehabil*. 2017;31:995-1004.

4. Nagi S. Disability concepts revisited: implications for prevention. In: Pope AM, Tarlov AR, eds. *Disability in America: Toward a National Agenda for Prevention*. Washington, DC: National Academy Press; 1991:309-327.

5. Pope AM, Tarlov AR. *Disability in America*. Washington, DC: National Academy Press; 1991.

6. World Health Organization. *International Classification of Functioning, Disability and Health: ICF*. Geneva, Switzerland: World Health Organization; 2001.

7. World Health Organization. ICF 2017 update. https://www.who.int/classifications/network/en/. Published 2017. Accessed December 17, 2018.

8. World Health Organization. ICF checklist version 2.1a. https://www.who.int/classifications/icf/icfchecklist.pdf. Published 2003. Accessed December 17, 2018.

9. World Health Organization. International Classification of Health Interventions. https://www.who.int/classifications/ichi/en/. Published 2018. Accessed December 17, 2018.

10. Jette AM. Toward a common language for function, disability, and health. *Phys Ther*. 2006;86:726-734.

11. American Physical Therapy Association. APTA endorses World Health Organization ICF model. http://www.apta.org/Media/Releases/APTA/2008/7/8/. Published 2008. Accessed December 17, 2018.

12. Selb M, Escorpizo R, Kostanjsek N, Stucki G, Ustun B, Cieza A. A guide on how to develop an International Classification of Functioning, Disability and Health Core Set. *Eur J Phys Rehabil Med*. 2015;51:105-117.

13. World Health Organization. ICF core sets. https://www.icf-core-sets.org/. Published 2012. Accessed December 17, 2017.

14. American Physical Therapy Association. *Guide to Physical Therapist Practice 3.0*. http://guidetoptpractice.apta.org. Accessed March 29, 2019.

15. Redgate N, Foto M. Pay by the rules: avoid Medicare audits and reduce payment denials with a sound strategy and proper documentation. *Physical Therapy Products*. 2003;October/November:28-30.

CHAPTER 2

Reasons for Documenting in Physical Therapy

Mia L. Erickson, PT, EdD

CHAPTER OUTLINE

- Record Patient/Client Management
- Communicate With Others
- Demonstrate Clinical Problem Solving
- Support Reimbursement
- Meet Reasonable and Necessary Criteria
    - Medical Necessity
    - Skilled Care
- Facilitate Administrative Duties
- Serve as a Legal Record of Care

CHAPTER OBJECTIVES

Upon completion of this chapter, the reader will be able to:

1. List reasons for documenting in physical therapy
2. List components of patient/client management that are included in documentation
3. Explain how other providers use physical therapy documentation
4. Explain how documentation demonstrates clinical problem solving
5. Explain the physical therapist assistant's role in the clinical decision-making process
6. Examine the relationship between reimbursement and documentation
7. Describe reasonable and necessary criteria and skilled care
8. Differentiate between skilled care and maintenance therapy
9. List situations when maintenance therapy can be considered skilled care
10. Describe how documentation can be used in legal matters

Erickson ML, Utzman RR, McKnight RS.
Physical Therapy Documentation: From Examination to Outcome,
Third Edition (pp 7-14).
© 2020 Taylor & Francis Group.

KEY TERMS

maintenance
reasonable and necessary
reimbursement
skilled care
third-party payer

KEY ABBREVIATIONS

CMS

TABLE 2-1

REASONS FOR DOCUMENTING IN PHYSICAL THERAPY

Record patient/client management

Communicate with others

Demonstrate clinical problem solving

Support reimbursement

Meet reasonable and necessary criteria including demonstrating medical necessity and proof of skilled care provided

Facilitate administrative duties

Serve as a legal record of care

RECORD PATIENT/CLIENT MANAGEMENT

Our documentation serves as a record of patient/client management (Table 2-1). In documenting patient/client management, the physical therapist creates and provides evidence of the episode of care that begins with the physical therapy referral (may be self-referral if the patient accesses physical therapy through direct access) and concludes with the discharge summary, or the summary of the final outcome. The documentation includes all relevant patient data, the physical therapist's assessment of the patient's condition, all interventions provided, and other information relevant to the patient's care. It helps the physical therapist who created the record to remember important patient data, interventions, and plans. The law requires health care providers to maintain a record of health care provided to patients. Accurate documentation is also an ethical responsibility, as outlined in the Code of Ethics for the Physical Therapist.[1]

COMMUNICATE WITH OTHERS

Records of patient/client data and care provided are important to other individuals involved in the patient's management, and these records serve as a useful means of communication. Other health care providers including physicians, nurses, occupational and speech therapists, and case managers are often interested in a patient's status, and these individuals often need to refer to the physical therapy documentation. For example, in an inpatient hospital setting, a physician might be interested in how safely and independently a patient can ambulate when deciding whether to send the patient home. Nurses might be interested in a patient's ability to transfer in and out of bed, and case managers often need to identify equipment needs or return-to-work status. Therefore, documenting patient data serves as a useful tool for facilitating communication across disciplines.

In addition to communication with nonphysical therapy providers, documentation serves as a reference for other physical therapy providers who work with your patients in your absence. It is important that the documentation provides accurate and clear information for the individual assuming the care of the patient. Clearly written notes help those treating in your absence provide appropriate and consistent care much more efficiently.

Transfer of physical therapy services from one setting to another (eg, acute care to home health or acute care to inpatient rehabilitation) is also quite common, and well-written notes can facilitate continuity of care across settings. Transfer of care can also happen between 2 physical therapists and between physical therapists and physical therapist assistants. A physical therapist assistant assuming the care of the patient relies on the physical therapist's documentation to provide information and direction. The physical therapist's documentation informs the physical therapist assistant regarding the patient's diagnosis, prognosis, and status so he or she knows what to expect and how to prepare for seeing the patient the first time. This might include things such as the level of assist needed for transfers and the assistive device used during gait. The physical therapist's documentation also alerts the physical therapist assistant to any precautions or restrictions such as weight-bearing status, allergies, or special indications or contraindications for treatment. The physical therapist assistant uses the physical therapist's documentation of the plan of care to provide the correct intervention(s) and progression.

DEMONSTRATE CLINICAL PROBLEM SOLVING

Physical therapy documentation should reflect and integrate clinical problem solving.[2] Any individual who provides aspects of patient/client management is responsible for ensuring the patient's record reflects clinical problem solving. Documentation that demonstrates clinical problem solving can improve communication between providers, support the rationale for services, demonstrate the unique skills provided to the patient, and thus help in securing reimbursement.

The medical record tells a story of the patient's physical therapy encounter. Any individual who does not know the patient should be able to read the physical therapy documentation and identify the patient's impairments, activity limitations, participation restrictions, contextual factors, interventions used, and the outcome. Another way to integrate clinical problem solving is to describe the effectiveness of the interventions provided. The following paragraphs describe ways a physical therapist can demonstrate clinical problem solving in the patient/client record.

During the initial examination:

- After collecting the initial subjective and objective examination data, the physical therapist creates a plan of care that draws the reader's attention to the patient's problems (eg, impairments, activity limitations, and participation restrictions) and outlines interventions aimed at reducing each. The prognosis and interventions are determined in a manner that considers relevant personal and environmental contextual factors, positive and negative. For example, a patient with poor endurance is treated with a program that includes cardiovascular activities aimed at building endurance, but if the patient has comorbidities, those would be documented and the prognosis and plan adjusted to accommodate.

At subsequent therapy sessions:

- Following the initial visit, relevant subjective and objective data are collected and recorded in interim notes. Subjective data collected during this phase can include (1) asking the patient about his or her response to a previous treatment, (2) inquiring about adherence with an exercise program, or (3) asking the patient if the treatment has improved his or her functional status. Objective data include relevant tests and measures that are consistent with those from the initial examination as well as any additional tests and measures that would be appropriate. Subjective remarks and results of tests and measures are compared between current and prior encounters. Changes in patient status, subjective or objective, are recorded in the documentation and brought to the reader's attention. For example, "The patient's active range of motion for left shoulder flexion improved from 90 to 120 degrees in 1 week" or "The patient ambulated 150' today with minimal assist of 1 to advance the left lower extremity compared to 50' with moderate assist of 2 1 week ago."

- Reductions in impairments brought on by the treatment that subsequently reduce activity limitations and participation restrictions should be described in detail. For example, you have been working with a patient following a total knee arthroplasty. The patient has been limited in his ability to don his shoes and sit comfortably in a chair because of limited active knee flexion (limited to 65 degrees). After 2 weeks of exercise, the patient's knee range of motion has improved 35 degrees (now 100 degrees). As a result, the patient is now able to sit more comfortably in a chair and don his shoes without assistance. In this scenario, one documents how the interventions have helped in reducing impairments and improving function (eg, "Range of motion exercises have helped in increasing knee flexion from 65 to 100 degrees, and now Mr. Smith is able to sit more comfortably and don his shoes independently").

- Adjustments to the interventions occur based on the patient's status, either positively or negatively. Adjustments made are supported by the clinical findings reported in the documentation. A physical therapist assistant working with the patient may carry out these adjustments as long as the changes are within the current plan of care and are permissible by law for the physical therapist assistant's scope of practice. If changes fall outside the plan of care, then the physical therapist is responsible for making the adjustments and updating the plan of care.

Integrating clinical problem solving into documentation is important but easily overlooked. Ongoing, comparative, and descriptive documentation of subjective remarks, objective findings, and functional changes tell the story of the patient's response to treatment. Referencing and making comparisons with prior data make it easy for a reader to follow the clinical problem-solving process and identify progress or a lack thereof.

SUPPORT REIMBURSEMENT

In the 1960s, medical records existed to (1) provide a legal record of care, (2) facilitate communication among health care providers, and (3) serve as a source of information for clinical research.[3] In the 1970s, documentation became a reimbursement requirement by government agencies such as Medicare and Medicaid. Medicare began requiring rehabilitation facilities not only to maintain documentation but also to submit records to be reviewed by Medicare auditors. Auditors reviewed documentation to determine if physical therapy services provided to Medicare beneficiaries met the requirements for reimbursement.[3] Today, documentation is a requirement for all third-party payers. It meets payment objectives by supporting what was billed.[4] Payers continue to conduct audits to determine if the documentation supports the need for the services provided and billed.

To support reimbursement, documentation should not only provide a record of what was billed on a particular date of service, but also it should focus on the rationale for services provided.[5] Consider the following example:

> You are working in a skilled nursing facility and you receive a phone call from an insurance agency that some of your billing procedures have triggered an external audit. They are asking that you submit documentation from 15 patient charts for dates of service January 1 through June 30 from the previous year. The plan is for the agency to review the documentation and determine if it supports the payments you received for these patients' claims. If documentation DOES NOT support services billed, then the facility where you are working will be required to pay back the money already reimbursed.

Audits can be devastating for facilities, managers, and therapists. They can also be financially draining. You can see from this example the importance of adequate documentation that supports what was billed in the event of an audit.

In addition to justifying interventions billed, especially in the event of an audit, documentation helps support the need for further physical therapy services. Documentation that shows patient improvement can help in securing necessary visits.

> You are a physical therapist working in a small, outpatient private practice. For the last 6 weeks, you have been working with a 35-year-old man who was recently involved in a motorcycle accident. In the accident, he sustained a mild concussion and multiple left lower extremity fractures. Initially, he was unable to bear weight through the extremity and required a wheelchair for mobility. He had significant loss in range of motion and strength. He was unable to perform independent self-care, normal home and community mobility including ambulation, or his usual work activities. Since the initial visit, he has been making excellent progress and is now able to walk using one crutch, weight bearing as tolerated, and has resumed most of his normal activities of daily living. After seeing him for 14 visits, it is brought to your attention that his insurance requires authorization for visits occurring after the initial 15. In order to have additional therapy services approved, you must submit adequate documentation showing evidence of (1) patient progress and (2) justification for continuing treatment.

The continuation of physical therapy benefits for this patient may be based largely on how well you have objectively documented his improvement and how well you can justify that additional services are necessary for his condition. As a therapist, it is difficult to stay abreast of documentation requirements for reimbursement, especially when you work with a diverse mix of payers. Payer documentation requirements can also be somewhat vague and difficult to find and translate into clinical practice. The American Physical Therapy Association provides guidelines for physical therapy documentation.[6,7] The Centers for Medicare & Medicaid Services (CMS) has also provided documentation requirements for those working with Medicare beneficiaries in various settings.[8] These resources can help physical therapy providers keep patient records that support services provided in the event of an audit and are appropriate for securing reimbursement or additional services.

MEET REASONABLE AND NECESSARY CRITERIA

Clinical documentation serves to justify that care provided to patients is reasonable and necessary. The phrase "reasonable and necessary" originated from language describing benefits covered by Medicare. However, in clinical documentation, it is often difficult to articulate *how* services are reasonable and necessary. Nevertheless, it is expected to be an integral part of documentation in the event of an audit or when requesting additional services. CMS published the following conditions that should be met in order for services to be considered reasonable and necessary in the outpatient therapy setting[9]:

- The services shall be considered under accepted standards of medical practice to be a specific and effective treatment for the patient's condition.

- The services provided to the patient are at a level of complexity and sophistication that can be provided only by a therapist or assistant under appropriate supervision (see "skilled care" in next section). Services that do not require performance or supervision by a therapist are not skilled and are not covered under the reasonable and necessary therapy services, even if they are performed by qualified personnel. If the contractor determines services were not furnished under proper supervision, the claim will be denied.

- Although the patient's medical condition is a valid factor in considering whether services are skilled, a beneficiary's diagnosis or prognosis should never be the sole factor in deciding that a service is or is not skilled. The key issue is whether the skills of a therapist are needed to treat the illness or injury or whether the services can be carried out by nonskilled personnel.

- An expectation exists that the patient's condition will improve significantly in a reasonable (and generally predictable) period of time or the services must be necessary for the establishment of a safe and effective maintenance program required in connection with a specific disease state. In the case of a progressive degenerative disease, services may be necessary to determine the need for assistive or adaptive equipment and/or to establish a program to maximize patient function.

- The amount, frequency, and duration of the services must be reasonable under accepted standards of practice in the local area or according to state or national therapy associations and guidelines.

These criteria are used for general purposes, but, since their implementation, CMS has provided more specific criteria for various physical therapy settings.[9,10] For example, in inpatient rehabilitation facilities, the following must be met at the time of admission[10]:

- The patient must require active and ongoing therapeutic intervention of multiple disciplines (physical therapy, occupational therapy, speech-language pathology, or prosthetics/orthotics), one of which must be physical therapy or occupational therapy.

- The patient must generally require an intensive rehabilitation therapy program; under current industry standards, this generally consists of 3 hours of therapy per day at least 5 days per week, or in well-documented cases may consist of 15 hours within a consecutive 7-day period, beginning with the date of admission.

- The patient must reasonably be expected to actively participate in, and benefit significantly from, the intensive rehabilitation therapy program. The patient need not be expected to achieve complete independence in the domain of self-care nor be expected to return to his or her prior level of functioning in order to meet this standard.

- The patient must require physician supervision by a rehabilitation physician, defined as a licensed physician with specialized training and experience in inpatient rehabilitation. The physician must conduct face-to-face visits with the patient at least 3 days per week throughout the patient's stay in the inpatient rehabilitation facility to assess the patient both medically and functionally as well as to modify the course of treatment as needed to maximize the patient's capacity to benefit from the rehabilitation process.

- The patient must require an intensive and coordinated interdisciplinary approach to providing rehabilitation.

Other third-party payers besides Medicare may also use these conditions. It is the therapist's responsibility to stay abreast of conditions set forth by payers for what is considered reasonable and necessary.

Proving that treatment is reasonable and necessary in documentation can be difficult and should be done on a case-by-case basis beginning with the consideration of data from the initial examination and the creation of the intervention plan, or plan of care. Physical therapists should consider the best available evidence for the given pathology,

illness, or injury; and the specific skills that are needed to address the impairments, activity limitations, and participation restrictions identified in the data. Integrating concepts showing good clinical decision making is also necessary. At regular intervals throughout the episode of care, the physical therapist should document to provide proof that interventions *continue* to be reasonable and necessary. To do this, the therapist summarizes changes brought on by the interventions, provides a list of remaining deficits, and describes the need for continuing services.

When the individual is not responding to treatment as expected, justifying reasonable and necessary care is more challenging. The therapist must discern the reason why the patient is not responding. Perhaps the intervention should be adjusted or there are contextual factors complicating the situation, such as a complicating diagnosis or social situation. Another consideration is that the patient has reached his or her maximum potential for improvement. Whatever the reason, if the therapist chooses to continue, the documentation must be able to support that ongoing services satisfy the reasonable and necessary criteria.

Medical Necessity

A similar phrase used in practice is "medical necessity" or "medically necessary." CMS defines medically necessary as health care services or supplies needed to diagnose or treat an illness, injury, condition, disease, or its symptoms and that meet accepted standards of medicine.[11] Medical necessity is only one aspect of the reasonable and necessary criteria. To document medical necessity, the therapist documents the scientific rationale or the purpose for a particular treatment. This will be discussed throughout the text. Look at the following examples that show the rationale for the treatment:

- The patient requires prolonged passive stretch to increase tissue elasticity and restore range of motion, or

- The patient requires ultrasound for deep tissue heating to improve tissue elasticity before stretching, or

- The patient requires gait training to improve independence, safety, and endurance.

Skilled Care

Another important aspect of the reasonable and necessary criteria that warrants further discussion is proving the need for "skilled services" or "skilled care." Clinical documentation should provide proof that care provided to a patient is "skilled." Skilled services are those that have inherent complexity that, for safety and/or effectiveness, must be carried out *only* by or under the supervision of a skilled therapist to achieve patient safety and the medically desired outcome.[10] This intervention may also require the unique judgment of a trained individual. Although the patient's medical condition or pathology is a factor in deciding whether skilled services are needed, neither the diagnosis nor the prognosis should ever be the sole factor in determining whether a patient needs the skills of a therapist.[9] Rather, the need for the skills of a therapist is determined by all factors surrounding the patient's condition and the desired outcomes.

In the clinical documentation, to provide proof of skilled care, the therapist documents or describes the specific "skill" provided to a patient during the intervention or functional task. Consider the following 2 statements from a patient record and determine which one specifically describes the skills provided by the therapist:

1. The patient ambulated 50' with a wide-based quad cane and minimal assist × 1.
2. The patient ambulated 50' with a wide-based quad cane with minimal assist × 1, which included manual assist and tactile cues to facilitate swing and prevent toe drag.

The second example shows how the unique skills of the therapist were used in the session and demonstrates the need for skilled gait training. Documentation must show that provider services are medically necessary and skilled.[5]

Some services are considered palliative or maintenance. Maintenance services are those that are routine, promote the general health of the patient, "maintain" the patient's present status, and do not require the unique, complex, or sophisticated skills of a physical therapist for safety and/or effectiveness.[9] Maintenance can be performed by the patient or by an unlicensed individual, such as the family member or caregiver who has received training from a skilled professional.

However, there are times when maintenance services are considered skilled care. These include the following[9]:

- When the physical therapist or physical therapist assistant works with the patient and/or family to establish and provide instruction in a home exercise program before discharge from a facility
- When a physical therapist evaluates a patient and establishes a home exercise/maintenance program when no other services are provided (eg, a patient with osteoarthritis is referred to physical therapy for examination and establishment of an aquatic therapy program; following the examination, the physical therapist works with the patient for 3 sessions to increase the patient's independence in performing the aquatic program)
- When the patient's safety may be jeopardized as in cases in which the patient has a complex, unpredictable medical situation, multiple comorbidities complicating his or her situation, or the result of the situation or intervention is unpredictable. This rule may apply to a patient who has a recent or unstable fracture and requires passive range of motion exercises. In some situations, passive range of motion exercises may be considered routine, or maintenance, but due to the fracture, the patient requires the treatment to be performed by a licensed therapist.

Although in many cases the assumption for patient improvement exists, this is not always the case. Consider patients with chronic or degenerative conditions and those individuals who have late-stage palliative care diagnoses.[12] These individuals may require physical therapy services to maintain or slow a decline, and based on CMS standards, improvement is not a requirement for reimbursement for Medicare beneficiaries.[12] In fact, the decision for payment is based on whether the treatment is medically necessary and requires the skills of a therapist. The burden of proof for establishing medical necessity in the documentation rests on the physical therapist or physical therapist assistant.[12] In order to meet documentation standards in this situation, authors have emphasized the need for statements referencing why the treatments are required, the anticipated detrimental effects if the treatments were not received, and statements that show proof that the treatment is needed and cannot be carried out by nonlicensed personnel.[12]

FACILITATE ADMINISTRATIVE DUTIES

In some clinics or health care systems, administrators use the medical record or physical therapy documentation to perform necessary administrative tasks. The medical record informs quality improvement activities, helps in determining or comparing the cost-effectiveness of services, and serves as data for marketing and growth. In acute care hospitals, skilled nursing units, and inpatient rehabilitation settings, administrators use the medical record to identify the case mix groups in the facility. The case mix describes the characteristics of the patients admitted to a particular unit or facility. Physical therapy documentation also aids in our ability to analyze patient data to determine best practice.[4] Physical therapists are beginning to use data registries created when clinical data are pulled from the electronic health record into a database. These registries serve as data sets for large-scale research studies.

SERVE AS A LEGAL RECORD OF CARE

Medical records are legal documents, and any entries made into the medical record become part of that legal document. For this reason, it is important your documentation is accurate, legible, and depicts the patient's condition and the intervention appropriately and completely. Be aware that a patient's medical records can be subpoenaed and used as evidence in a variety of legal matters. These include motor vehicle accidents, worker's compensation or disability claims, and malpractice suits brought against you or other health care providers.

In malpractice lawsuits, documentation is the clinician's first line of defense.[13] Notes that are "clear, objective, thorough, and relevant make plaintiff's allegations of negligence more difficult to prove."[14(p2)] Good documentation can prevent a lawsuit, but poor documentation can be "powerful evidence in support of a suit, even when the accusations are frivolous."[15(p30)] Consider the following as a rule of thumb: if it is not documented, it did not happen. Following the guidelines for documentation in this text, recommendations set forth by the American Physical Therapy Association, state and federal laws, government agency requirements (eg, Medicare and Medicaid), and facility policies can help to protect you if you become involved in a malpractice lawsuit. Legal and ethical issues regarding documentation are described more in the next chapter.

REVIEW QUESTIONS

1. List the reasons for documenting in physical therapy.

2. What aspects of patient/client management are included in the documentation?

3. Explain how a clinician's clinical problem solving should be reflected in his or her documentation.

4. What other individuals may be reviewing documentation written by a physical therapist?

5. What information does a physical therapist assistant gather from the physical therapist's documentation?

6. How is documentation tied with reimbursement?

7. What are the criteria for determining if an intervention is reasonable and necessary?

8. How can a physical therapist demonstrate medical necessity in the documentation? How can a physical therapist demonstrate that a particular service was "skilled"?

9. Give 2 examples of when maintenance therapy would be considered "skilled."

10. What are the therapists' requirements for documenting on a patient/client who has a chronic or degenerative condition but requires skilled services?

APPLICATION EXERCISES

Read through the following scenarios and answer the following question for each. What should the physical therapist consider when deciding whether or not to discharge the patient from his or her caseload?

1. You are working with a patient in a nursing home who has severe Alzheimer's disease. Every afternoon, you take her for a walk through the hallways and around the building. She demonstrates weakness in her right ankle, and there is a foot slap during the contact phase of gait. She can control it if given verbal cueing. You have been working with her for a month and you are not seeing any follow-through from one session to the next, and she has not progressed her distance or assistance needed in the last 2 weeks.

2. You have been working for a home health agency in the evenings to make some extra money. The patient you are currently seeing has not shown improvement in the last 2 weeks, and the exercise program could be carried out by a family member. She is an 85-year-old woman with Parkinson's disease who lives with her daughter. You are considering discharge when one day, the patient's daughter tells you that her mother enjoys having you come to the house, and they really believe that you are helping.

3. You are working in a skilled nursing unit, and you are assigned a patient who requires maximum assist for transfers due to a femur fracture and non–weight-bearing restrictions.

4. You are working in an outpatient physical therapy clinic with a patient who has a frozen shoulder. She has been participating in therapy for 6 weeks. During that time, she has made a substantial amount of progress. Over the last 2 weeks, her range of motion has started to plateau, and she has resumed 90% of her functional activities. The patient attends therapy twice a week for passive stretching.

5. You are working on gait training with a patient who had a right cerebrovascular accident and has resultant left hemiplegia. While ambulating, you provide tactile and verbal cueing to the quadriceps to achieve full knee extension in late swing. The patient can respond to your cues about 50% of the time. This has improved over the last week, and the patient requires less assistance than during the initial examination.

REFERENCES

1. American Physical Therapy Association House of Delegates. Code of Ethics for the Physical Therapist. HOD S06-09-07-12. https://www.apta.org/uploadedFiles/APTAorg/About_Us/Policies/Ethics/CodeofEthics.pdf. Accessed March 29, 2019.

2. Osborne J. Documentation helps clinicians help people. *GeriNotes*. 2018;25(3):16-18.

3. Inaba M, Jones SLL. Medical documentation for third-party payers. *Phys Ther*. 1977;57:791-794.

4. Evans WK, Elrod M. Compliance matters: creating a written portrait. *PT in Motion*. 2018;10(9):6-9.

5. Evans WK. Complaince matters: the keys to effective documentation. *PT in Motion*. 2016;8:8-12.

6. American Physical Therapy Association. Guidelines: physical therapy documentation of patient/client management. BOD G03-05-16-41. https://www.apta.org/uploadedFiles/APTAorg/About_Us/Policies/Practice/DocumentationPatientClientManagement.pdf. February 18, 2020.

7. American Physical Therapy Association. Defensible documentation. http://www.apta.org/DefensibleDocumentation/. Published July 2010. Accessed February 18, 2020.

8. Centers for Medicare and Medicaid Services. *Medicare Benefit Policy Manual*. Publication no. 100-02. https://www.cms.gov/Regulations-and-Guidance/Guidance/Manuals/Internet-Only-Manuals-IOMs-Items/CMS012673. Published June 2006. Accessed February 18, 2020.

9. Centers for Medicare and Medicaid Services. Medicare Benefit Policy Manual. Publication no. 100-02. Chapter 15. https://www.cms.gov/Regulations-and-Guidance/Guidance/Manuals/Downloads/bp102c15.pdf. Published July 12, 2019. Accessed February 18, 2020.

10. Centers for Medicare and Medicaid Services. Medicare Benefit Policy Manual. Publication no. 100-02. Chapter 1. https://www.cms.gov/Regulations-and-Guidance/Guidance/Manuals/Downloads/bp102c01.pdf. Published March 10, 2017. Accessed February 18, 2020.

11. Centers for Medicare and Medicaid Services. Glossary. https://www.cms.gov/apps/glossary/default.asp. Published 2006. Accessed April 10, 2019.

12. Wilson CM, Boright L. Documenting medical necessity for palliative care and degenerative or chronic conditions. *Rehabil Oncol*. 2017;35:153-156.

13. Schunk CRR. Liability awareness. Advice for the new physical therapist: here are some keys to avoiding risk once you've made the transition from student to practitioner. *PT Magazine*. 2001;9(11):24-26.

14. Lewis DK. Lessons from COURT. *HPSO Risk Advisor*. 2000;3(2):1-2.

15. Lewis DK. Do the write thing: document everything. *PT Magazine*. 2002;10(7):30-34.

CHAPTER 3

Ethical, Legal, and Regulatory Issues in Physical Therapy Documentation

Ralph R. Utzman, PT, MPH, PhD

CHAPTER OUTLINE

- Law, Regulation, and Policy
- Informed Consent
- Malpractice and Risk Management
- Patient Safety and Quality of Care
- Confidentiality
- Reimbursement, Fraud, and Abuse

CHAPTER OBJECTIVES

Upon completion of this chapter, the reader will be able to:

1. Compare and contrast law, regulation, and policy
2. Describe how APTA's Code of Ethics for the Physical Therapist addresses documentation-related issues such as informed consent, confidentiality, reimbursement, fraud, and abuse
3. Define informed consent
4. Discuss how documentation serves as a risk management tool
5. Describe the function of the medical record as a communication tool to improve patient safety and quality of care
6. Describe the purpose of incident reports and identify how incident reports should be filed
7. Describe how HIPAA safeguards patient privacy

Erickson ML, Utzman RR, McKnight RS.
Physical Therapy Documentation: From Examination to Outcome,
Third Edition (pp 15-21).
© 2020 Taylor & Francis Group.

KEY TERMS

abuse
claims review
critical incident
fraud
Health Insurance Portability and
Accountability Act (HIPAA)
incident report
informed consent
practice acts
preauthorization
regulations
utilization review

KEY ABBREVIATIONS

APTA
HIPAA

The previous chapter described the clinical problem-solving skills physical therapists use to provide patient care. To solve patient problems, physical therapists access, record, and transmit a wide variety of patients' medical, personal, and social information. The primary vehicle for this information is the medical record, which is itself a legal document. Therefore, physical therapist practice requires careful attention to ethical principles and compliance with laws and regulations related to documentation and the medical record.

This chapter introduces readers to ethical, legal, and regulatory issues related to clinical documentation. This chapter is not intended as a substitute for professional legal advice. Many health care facilities employ or retain licensed attorneys to assist with managing legal risks associated with providing health care. Other facilities, as well as therapists in private practice, can obtain legal advice from the insurance company from whom they purchase malpractice/liability coverage. Many organizations have compliance officers or departments that assist health care providers in understanding and following current regulations. Readers are urged to seek advice from one of these sources when confronted with specific questions in clinical practice.

LAW, REGULATION, AND POLICY

Laws are governmental statements of what we must do. They are developed by votes of Congress, state legislatures, or county/municipal governments. Laws can also result from court cases in which a decision by a judge or jury sets a precedent for future cases. Laws often delegate oversight of a law to a government agency or regulatory body. This government agency may then write regulations, or rules, that state how the intent of the law is to be carried out. Such regulations typically carry the force of law.

For example, consider state laws that govern physical therapist practice. In all 50 states, laws exist that define what physical therapy is and who can practice physical therapy. These laws, which are enacted by state legislatures, are commonly known as physical therapy practice acts. In most states, these practice acts include provisions for a licensure board, which is a government agency that oversees practice of physical therapy. In turn, the licensure board may write regulations that further describe parameters of practice. If a therapist fails to comply with either the practice act or regulations, the licensing board may suspend or revoke the therapist's license to practice.

Although laws and regulations are written by the government and its agencies, policies are rules written by nongovernmental organizations. Such organizations include professional associations (eg, the American Physical Therapy Association [APTA]) or accrediting bodies (eg, The Joint Commission). Health care organizations, like hospitals and clinics, also develop policies that govern their employees. A primary purpose of organizational policy is to standardize the actions and behaviors of members of that organization. Organizational policies can also serve to communicate the values and philosophies that guide members' behaviors.

APTA has several policies related to the documentation of physical therapy care. The APTA's Guidelines for Physical Therapy Documentation[1] outlines the profession's standards for documentation. The guidelines are rooted in a broader APTA document, the Code of Ethics for the Physical Therapist.[2]

The Code of Ethics for the Physical Therapist consists of 8 principles that are broad statements of physical therapists' responsibilities.[2] Each of the 8 principles includes 2 or more additional statements that further define therapists' responsibilities in that particular area. Out of the 8 main principles, 5 specifically address issues related to documentation and communication with other health care personnel. The following sections of this chapter address specific ethical and legal issues related to documentation, with references to the Code of Ethics and key regulations as applicable.

INFORMED CONSENT

Informed consent refers to the right of the patient to make his or her own decisions about the care he or she receives. Principle 2C of the Code of Ethics states, "Physical therapists shall provide the information necessary to allow patients ... to make informed decisions about physical therapy care ...."[2] In order to make a decision, the patient needs to know the examination results, what treatment is being recommended, the potential benefits, costs, and risks of that treatment, and what alternatives exist. The best way for a physical therapist to accomplish this is to discuss each of these elements with the patient and then document the outcome of the discussion. The APTA's Guidelines for Physical Therapy Documentation[1] recommend this documentation be included in the prognosis and plan of care. For example, the physical therapist could include the following statement in a plan of care:

> The patient and therapist discussed the recommended treatment plan, including potential risks of the intervention and how they will be minimized. The patient's questions regarding potential muscle soreness were answered, and the patient agreed with the plan.

Note that the statement should be customized according to the plan of care and the patient's response.

Many health care facilities ask patients to sign formal consent forms. The length and scope of these forms vary by facility and procedure. For example, many facilities ask patients to sign brief "consent to treat" forms when patients register for care. For surgical procedures and other high-risk services, facilities will use more extensive forms that include fields for each element of consent (eg, test results, recommended treatment, benefits, risks, and alternatives). Such forms should be viewed as cues to guide and document ongoing dialogue with the patient and not be used as a substitute for such discussions. Simply put, informed consent is NOT a form.

Even though physical therapy care is typically conservative and presents low risks to patients compared with surgery and medications, no treatment is completely risk free. Suppose that a therapist performs a stretching technique with a patient following tendon repair surgery. Even though an appropriate amount of time has elapsed since the surgery and the therapist has communicated with the patient's surgeon regarding the planned treatment, there is still a small chance that stretching may cause the repaired tendon to rupture. The therapist should discuss this, along with other treatment alternatives, with the patient and obtain consent before beginning the treatment. If the therapist provides the treatment and the repaired tendon is ruptured, the therapist may face a malpractice lawsuit. In such suits, a common claim is that the practitioner failed to obtain the patient's informed consent.[3] The therapist's best defense is careful documentation of the patient's clinical status,[3] the patient's informed consent to the stretching procedure, and the treatment and follow-up provided.

MALPRACTICE AND RISK MANAGEMENT

Any time a physical therapist provides care to a patient, the therapist is taking a legal risk. Malpractice lawsuits can result from a variety of issues. According to a report by a provider of malpractice/liability insurance,[4] the following are common allegations made against physical therapists:

- Improper management or treatment of the patient (eg, performing inappropriate treatment techniques)
- Improper performance of therapeutic exercise or manual therapy
- Failure to adequately supervise/monitor patients and support personnel
- Injury from modalities, such as hot packs or electrical stimulation
- Failure to perform appropriate tests/measures
- Injuries related to equipment and/or the care environment
- Improper behavior by the physical therapist

Many facilities employ risk managers, or utilize risk management committees or departments, whose responsibilities include minimizing potential risks for health care providers involved with patient/client management. In a private practice, the owner may serve as the risk manager. Besides providing training for clinicians on managing legal risks, these individuals or groups investigate complaints or concerns as they are brought forth, either by patients or providers. An important aspect of their investigation is examining the medical record and other available documentation. Good documentation is the cornerstone of good risk management, allowing risk managers to determine if quality care standards were met and how to avoid future risks.

Critical incidents include adverse events that result in patient harm as well as events that have the potential to cause harm but do not. For instance, a therapist may discover that an electrical stimulation machine is malfunctioning. Depending on the nature of the malfunction and when it was discovered, the patient may or may not suffer a burn. When an adverse event leads to patient injury, the therapist should record the objective facts regarding the incident in the medical record. These facts should include information regarding the injury, instructions given to the patient, communication of the incident with referring physicians or other health care providers, and any follow-up care provided to the patient.

Regardless of whether the incident harmed the patient, the therapist also should file an incident report. Incident reports are used to document patient safety "incidents" that may or may not have involved harm to the patient, "near misses" that were caught before the patient was placed in harm's way, and even unsafe conditions that increase the risk of patient harm.[5] Incident reports serve as a tool for improving care by identifying and investigating problems as they arise. Incident reports also provide an internal account in case legal action results from the adverse event.[6] Incident reports should be filed with your facility's risk management department or malpractice/liability insurer. In many organizations, traditional paper forms have been replaced with computerized systems to facilitate the reporting of incidents to the appropriate personnel.[7] Incident reports are used for administrative, quality improvement, and training purposes but are not a substitute for documentation in the medical record. In many states, incident reports are protected from release to the plaintiff's attorneys because they are considered internal quality improvement documents, privileged communication between the clinician and his or her attorney, or both.[6] Therefore, they should not be filed with or mentioned in the medical record.

PATIENT SAFETY AND QUALITY OF CARE

Principle 3 of the Code of Ethics states, "Physical therapists shall be accountable for making sound professional judgments."[2] Subitems included with this principle state that the physical therapist is independently responsible (rather than a referring physician or facility administrator) for the decisions he or she makes, that he or she is responsible for using the best scientific evidence to inform those decisions, and that clinical judgments must be communicated clearly with peers, subordinates (ie, physical therapist assistants), and other health care providers.[2] The primary method for communicating professional judgment and decisions is the medical record. The reader of physical therapy documentation should be able to identify the key findings of the physical therapy examination, the rationale for the plan of care, any precautions to be followed, and the patient's response to treatment.

The medical record was originally designed as a mechanism to remind the individual health care provider of the treatment provided to date. For physical therapists, accurately recalling the precautions, objective measurements, and exercise programs of multiple patients over time would be nearly impossible. Communicating this information to coworkers is critical. Consider the patients of a physical therapist who is called away from the clinic unexpectedly, and another therapist agrees to provide care for these patients in his or her absence. Without well-written medical records, the therapist filling in for the absent colleague would have no way to know what treatments had been provided previously, how the patients had responded, and what future treatments were planned. In this situation, the covering therapist would not be able to provide safe, effective treatment to the patients.

As the health care system has become increasingly specialized and complex, interprofessional communication and collaboration have been recognized as a core competency for all health care providers, including physical therapists.[8] Patients who have complex medical conditions, limitations, and precautions are frequently referred to physical therapy. Physical therapists are often supported by physical therapist assistants who provide elements of the plan of care with supervision from the physical therapist. In some settings and jurisdictions, the supervising physical therapist need not always be on-site while the assistant is providing treatment. In the absence of good documentation, communication of key information is likely to be missed, leading to poor quality of care and potential harm to the patient.

For example, consider the case of an older woman who has been admitted to a skilled nursing facility following surgical repair of a proximal femur fracture. The surgeon has referred the patient for physical therapy with a precaution that the patient should bear no more than 10% of her body weight on the involved lower extremity. Although the referral has been transmitted to the physical therapist, she neglects to document the weight-bearing precaution in her initial note and plan of care. Subsequent treatment sessions are provided by a physical therapist assistant. After several treatment sessions, the patient complains of increased hip and thigh pain in the involved extremity. The patient's family, concerned about the patient's increased pain, contacts the surgeon who orders a radiograph. The radiograph reveals that the surgical repair of the fracture has failed, and the patient requires further surgery. Because the physical therapist did not document the weight-bearing restriction in the plan of care, the medical record does not reflect professional judgment by the physical therapist. The therapist is responsible for the care provided by the assistant (Code of Ethics item 5C),[2] and with no clear documentation of the instructions provided to the assistant, the therapist may be found liable for the patient's poor clinical outcome.

Better patient outcomes can be achieved through improved documentation practices. Consider another patient with a similar diagnosis and referral. When admitted to the skilled nursing facility, the therapist carefully documents the postsurgical precautions. The patient is somewhat confused and has difficulty following instructions during the initial examination. The therapist documents this and carefully outlines a plan of care and instructions for the assistant. During subsequent treatments, the assistant notes the patient's difficulty to maintain the weight-bearing restrictions and appropriately limits progression of the patient's ambulation during treatment sessions. When reviewing the medical record before the next supervisory visit, the physical therapist notes the assistant's concerns as well as reports from nursing staff that the patient has been getting out of bed at night without assistance. The therapist notifies the surgeon and collaborates with the assistant and nursing staff regarding strategies to safely progress the patient's mobility. Together with the patient's family, the staff develops a plan to reduce the risk of the patient getting out of bed at night by herself. These plans and the patient's progress are carefully documented, and the patient gradually learns to use her walker safely without reinjuring herself. Although the patient stays in the facility for several days longer than initially expected, she returns home with her family without the need for further surgery.

CONFIDENTIALITY

Principle 2E of the Code of Ethics states that physical therapists must "... protect confidential patient/client information and may disclose confidential information ... only when allowed or as required by law."[2] This principle underscores the fact that physical therapists have access to a host of sensitive information about patients. Medical records may contain information about genetics, mental health, substance abuse, infectious diseases, and more. Some patients prefer to not share basic information, such as age or weight, even with close relatives. Medical records may include identifying data that can be exploited by identity thieves. Because medical records contain such sensitive data, they should be viewed as an extension of the individual and treated with the same respect and care expected by the patient.

Because of a series of high-profile breaches of patient confidentiality, the issue was included in the landmark federal law known as the Health Insurance Portability and Accountability Act (HIPAA) of 1996. Title I of HIPAA allows workers to maintain their insurance coverage when they change jobs. Title II focuses on preventing fraud and abuse and required the US Department of Health and Human Services to establish rules for safeguarding the privacy of patient's personal health information.

The final privacy rule developed by the US Department of Health and Human Services went into effect on April 14, 2003. Health care providers, health insurance plans, and health information clearinghouses are subject to the rule if they hold or transmit protected health information in any form—oral, written, facsimile, or electronic.[9] Protected health information includes all personal health information, including medical records and other identifiable health information.[9] Under the privacy rule, patients are granted several rights, including the following[9]:

- The right to read and get copies of their own medical records
- The right to make amendments to their own medical records
- The right to know who has access to their medical records
- The right to give written permission prior to disclosure of their personal health information

- The right to file a complaint when they believe their privacy is not being protected

The privacy rule allows health care providers to share information without written consent in circumstances that relate to routine care of the patient. Such circumstances would include providing information to other health care providers involved in the patient's care or providing copies of medical records to insurance companies for reimbursement purposes.[9,10] Such disclosures should provide only the minimum information necessary to accomplish the purpose.[9,11]

Under the HIPAA privacy rule, health care providers must obtain consent prior to releasing patients' protected health information for other reasons, such as marketing or research.[9] For instance, if a physical therapist or student is writing a case study on a patient, the author must obtain patient consent first. However, the material may be used without consent if it is first "deidentified." This means that any information that could potentially be used to identify the patient must be removed. The rule lists 18 elements that must be removed. In addition, the author would need to be sure that the patient could not be identified in any way from the remaining information.[10,12] The 18 elements that must be removed are listed in Table 3-1. These elements may be removed electronically or manually. Research protocols must be designed in ways that safeguard patient privacy, and these methods must be approved by an institutional review board.[9]

The privacy rule requires health care facilities to provide training related to patient privacy safeguards to their employees.[9] Facilities are also required to designate a privacy officer to oversee employee training and the overall implementation of privacy safeguards. Many states have laws regarding the privacy of personal health information. If the state law is more stringent than the HIPAA privacy rule, the state law supersedes HIPAA.

REIMBURSEMENT, FRAUD, AND ABUSE

As noted in the previous chapters, medical records are routinely used for insurance payment purposes. Medical records may be reviewed for preauthorization, or approval for payment prior to the delivery of nonemergency health care services. Medical records may be subject to utilization review during the course of care to make sure appropriate care is being provided. Claims review may be used after services are provided to compare the medical record with the final bill to make a final determination regarding whether or not services provided are to be reimbursed.

Principle 7B of the Code of Ethics states that "Physical therapists shall seek remuneration as is deserved and reasonable ...."[2] Furthermore, Principle 4A states that physical therapists shall "... provide truthful, accurate, and relevant

TABLE 3-1
DATA TO BE REMOVED TO DEIDENTIFY PATIENT RECORDS

1. Full name or last name and initials
2. All geographic identifiers of address smaller than the state
3. Dates related to the patient (eg, birth date, death date, and admission/discharge date) other than the year
4. Phone numbers
5. Facsimile numbers
6. Electronic mail addresses
7. Social Security numbers
8. Medical record numbers
9. Health insurance beneficiary numbers
10. Account numbers
11. Certificate/license numbers
12. Vehicle identifiers
13. Medical device identifiers (serial numbers)
14. Internet addresses (URLs)
15. Internet protocol (IP) address numbers
16. Fingerprints, retinal and voice prints, or other biometric data
17. Full-face photographs or similar images that could be used to identify the patient
18. Any other unique identifying number, code, or characteristic

Adapted from Guidance regarding methods for de-identification of protected health information in accordance with the HIPAA privacy rule. https://www.hhs.gov/hipaa/for-professionals/privacy/special-topics/de-identification/index.html#standard. Updated November 6, 2015. Accessed April 5, 2019.

A report from the Institute of Medicine[14] estimated fraud, waste, and abuse in the US health care system accounted for over $750 billion in 2009. Several federal laws have been enacted and used to combat this problem. For example, the False Claims Act, known as the *Lincoln Law*, has been applied to health care providers and entities that engage in fraud and abuse. Providers who knowingly submitted false claims (or should have known the claims were in error) can face severe financial penalties.[15] Other relevant laws include the Anti-Kickback Statute, the Physician Self-Referral Law, the Exclusion Statute, and the Civil Monetary Penalties Law.[15] In addition, many states have their own laws to combat insurance fraud and abuse.

In order to avoid accusations of abuse, physical therapists should stay abreast of and follow current billing and coding guidelines. According to the Code of Ethics Principle 7E, physical therapists have a duty to understand billing and coding for physical therapy services.[2] APTA has published 2 important resources to assist physical therapists in improving their documentation and avoiding fraud, waste, and abuse. Defensible Documentation for Patient/Client Management (www.apta.org/DefensibleDocumentation/) is a website that provides documentation tips, checklists, outlines, and examples that physical therapists can use to improve their documentation. The APTA Center for Integrity in Practice (www.integrity.apta.org) provides a downloadable primer, online continuing education courses, and best practices for preventing fraud, waste, and abuse.

As noted in the beginning of this chapter, documentation is inextricably linked to billing and reimbursement. In many ways, a complete, accurate, and truthful medical record is often considered to be the "itemized receipt" for health care services provided to the patient. Documentation must demonstrate that the services billed were provided to the patient, were medically necessary, and were skilled in nature. More detail on payment and reimbursement is provided in Chapter 12.

information and shall not make misleading representations."[2] Finally, Principle 5A states that physical therapists must comply with laws and regulations.[2] Taken together, the items from the code prohibit the physical therapist from engaging in reimbursement fraud and abuse. Insurance fraud can be defined as billing a third-party payer for services that were never provided or billing for an item or service that is reimbursed at a higher rate than the service that was actually provided.[13] Fraud is a crime and is punishable by law. Another improper billing procedure is abuse. Abuse occurs when a provider bills for items that are not covered or misuses billing codes.[13] Abuse differs from fraud in that fraud is intentional, whereas abuse often results from unintended billing errors or poor awareness of proper billing and coding procedures.

REVIEW QUESTIONS

1. What are the differences between laws, regulations, and policies? What are the similarities?
2. What functions do state boards of physical therapy serve?
3. Describe how the medical record serves as a tool for risk management.
4. What is informed consent? How should consent be documented in the medical record?
5. What are the purposes of the HIPAA privacy rule?
6. What types of occurrences should be documented on incident reports? How and where should incident reports be filed?

APPLICATION EXERCISES

1. Obtain copies of the physical therapy practice act (statutory law) and practice rules/regulations for your state. Review the documents and answer the following questions:

    a. What is the scope of practice of a physical therapist? A physical therapist assistant? Are there any limitations regarding what a physical therapist assistant is allowed to document compared with a physical therapist?

    b. What are the rules for supervising physical therapist assistants and other support personnel?

    c. Is a referral required for a patient to receive physical therapy services? If so, who may refer? If there are provisions for direct access (evaluation/treatment without referral), are there any limitations or restrictions?

    d. What rules apply to authenticating (signing) entries in the medical record? What initials should follow the physical therapist's name? If the therapist holds a Doctor of Physical Therapy degree, may he or she use this designator in the medical record? Is the therapist required to include his or her license number?

    e. What are the potential consequences for practice inconsistent with the practice act or rules/regulations?

2. Review your organization's policies and procedures for documentation. Do these policies coincide with APTA's Guidelines for Physical Therapy Documentation of Patient/Client Management?

3. Review your organization's policies for patient confidentiality and answer the following questions:

    a. How is the patient notified of his or her rights?

    b. How may a patient request copies of his or her medical record?

    c. How does the organization restrict access to the medical record?

    d. If a patient's confidentiality is breached, how would the facility respond? What sanctions would be taken against an employee who breaches patient confidentiality?

REFERENCES

1. American Physical Therapy Association. Guidelines: physical therapy documentation of patient/client management. http://www.apta.org/uploadedFiles/APTAorg/About_Us/Policies/Practice/DocumentationPatientClientManagement.pdf. Updated May 19, 2014. Accessed April 1, 2019.

2. American Physical Therapy Association. Code of ethics for the physical therapist. http://www.apta.org/uploadedFiles/APTAorg/About_Us/Policies/Ethics/CodeofEthics.pdf. Updated 2009. Accessed April 1, 2019.

3. Healthcare Providers Service Organization. Stay protected. In: *Perspectives*. Alexandria, VA: American Physical Therapy Association; 2016:4.

4. CNA and Healthcare Providers Service Organization. Physical therapy professional liability exposure: 2016 claim report update. http://image.exct.net/lib/fe6715707d6d017c7514/m/1/CNA_PT_CS_021116+SEC.pdf. Updated January 25, 2016. Accessed April 1, 2019.

5. Agency for Healthcare Research and Quality. Common formats. Patient Safety Organization Program website. https://www.pso.ahrq.gov/common. Accessed April 1, 2019.

6. Scott RW. Patient care record informed consent documentation issues. In: Scott RW, ed. *Legal, Ethical, and Practical Aspects of Patient Care Documentation*. 4th ed. Burlington, MA: Jones & Bartlett Learning; 2013:129-159.

7. Agency for Healthcare Research and Quality. Reporting patient safety events. Patient Safety Network website. https://psnet.ahrq.gov/primers/primer/13. Updated January 2019. Accessed April 1, 2019.

8. Interprofessional Education Collaborative. *Core Competencies for Interprofessional Collaborative Practice: 2016 Update*. Washington, DC: Interprofessional Education Collaborative; 2016.

9. US Department of Health & Human Services. Summary of the HIPAA Privacy Rule. Health information privacy website. https://www.hhs.gov/hipaa/for-professionals/privacy/laws-regulations/index.html. Updated July 26, 2013. Accessed April 1, 2019.

10. Gilliard KW. Are you hip to HIPAA? *PT in Motion*. 2019;11(1):8-10, 12.

11. US Department of Health & Human Services. Minimum necessary requirement. Health information privacy website. https://www.hhs.gov/hipaa/for-professionals/privacy/guidance/minimum-necessary-requirement/index.html. Updated July 26, 2013. Accessed April 1, 2019.

12. US Department of Health & Human Services. Guidance regarding methods for de-identification of protected health information in Accordance with the Health Insurance Portability and Accountability Act privacy rule. Health information privacy website. https://www.hhs.gov/hipaa/for-professionals/privacy/special-topics/de-identification/index.html#rationale. Updated November 6, 2015. Accessed April 1, 2019.

13. Centers for Medicare & Mediciaid Services. Glossary. https://www.cms.gov/apps/glossary/default.asp?Letter=F&Language=English. Updated May 14, 2006. Accessed April 1, 2019.

14. Institute of Medicine. *Best Care at Lower Cost: The Path to Continuously Learnign Health Care in America*. Washington, DC: The National Academies Press; 2013.

15. Office of the Inspector General. Roadmap for new physicians: fraud & abuse laws. US Department of Health & Human Services website. https://oig.hhs.gov/compliance/physician-education/01laws.asp. Accessed April 1, 2019.

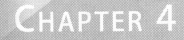

Documenting Patient/Client Management: An Overview

Mia L. Erickson, PT, EdD and Rebecca S. McKnight, PT, MS

CHAPTER OUTLINE

- Patient/Client Management
- Documenting the Initial Encounter
  - History, Systems Review, and Tests and Measures
  - Diagnosis, Prognosis, and Intervention
- Documenting Interim Visits
- Documenting Discharge

CHAPTER OBJECTIVES

Upon completion of this chapter, the reader will be able to:
1. Describe components of the Patient/Client Management Model
2. List requirements for documenting the initial visit with a patient/client
3. Differentiate between the examination and evaluation according to the Patient/Client Management Model
4. Realize the differing definitions for "evaluation"
5. Realize the importance of documenting impairments, activity limitations, participation restrictions, and contextual factors
6. Differentiate between the medical diagnosis and the diagnosis established by the physical therapist
7. List information that should be included in the initial plan of care
8. Compare and contrast interim (or treatment) notes and progress reports
9. Describe the role of the discharge note or summary

Erickson ML, Utzman RR, McKnight RS.
*Physical Therapy Documentation: From Examination to Outcome,
Third Edition* (pp 23-31).
© 2020 Taylor & Francis Group.

KEY TERMS

assessment
daily note
discharge
discharge note
discontinuation
evaluation
examination
interim note
Patient/Client Management Model
progress note (report)
reassessment
re-evaluation
treatment note

KEY ABBREVIATIONS

CMS

PATIENT/CLIENT MANAGEMENT

The *Guide to Physical Therapist Practice*[1] defines the role of the physical therapist with regard to patient care through the Patient/Client Management Model. The Patient/Client Management Model consists of 6 elements, or components, that include examination, evaluation, diagnosis, prognosis, intervention, and outcome.[1] The outcome is the result of the intervention. During the initial patient/client encounter, the physical therapist performs and documents the initial examination and evaluation. The Patient/Client Management Model differentiates examination from evaluation in that the *examination* is the process that includes taking a patient history, performing a systems review, and performing specific tests and measures, whereas the *evaluation* is a thought process that includes integration and interpretation of the data collected, determination of a diagnosis and prognosis amenable to physical therapy management, and development of a plan of care. The Patient/Client Management Model clearly differentiates between the terms and processes of examination and evaluation, although clinically the terms are often used synonymously. Additionally, in the clinical setting, the 2 processes are often collectively referred to as "the initial evaluation." Furthermore, the Centers for Medicare & Medicaid Services (CMS) defines evaluation as follows[2(p154)]:

A separately payable comprehensive service provided by a clinician, that requires professional skills to make clinical judgments about conditions for which services are indicated based on objective measurements and subjective evaluations of patient performance and functional abilities. Evaluation is warranted for a new diagnosis or when a condition is treated in a new setting. These evaluative judgments are essential to development of the plan of care, including goals and the selection of interventions.

Because there are many definitions for the terms *examination* and *evaluation*, there is basis for confusion. In order to be consistent with the *Guide to Physical Therapist Practice* and the Patient/Client Management Model, throughout this text, we refer to *examination* as the process of collecting patient/client-related data and *evaluation* as the process of clinical decision making that occurs following the examination.

DOCUMENTING THE INITIAL ENCOUNTER

History, Systems Review, and Tests and Measures

At the onset of the initial encounter, the physical therapist performs the examination by taking the patient/client history, performing a systems review, and performing specific tests and measures and documenting the results. The patient/client history comes from the patient or client, a family member, or caregiver and forms the subjective portion of the examination. It includes demographic information and information about the present illness or condition such as the mechanism and date of injury, chief or current complaints, and the impact on functional status including activities and participation. Questions asked during the history-taking portion of the examination also include those related to the patient's social history, work or employment history, growth or development, living environment, general health status, social and health habits (past and current), family history, medications, and other clinical or diagnostic tests.[1] During the history, the physical therapist should also ask questions to glean information regarding the body systems that can be helpful in differentiating musculoskeletal conditions from serious medical conditions that require immediate referral to another provider. Self-report general health and screening questionnaires can also aid in gathering information related to the patient's body systems. Both the *Guide to Physical Therapist Practice*[1] and the Guidelines for Physical Therapy Documentation of Patient/Client Management[3] provide examples of typical data gathered during the history-taking portion of the examination. More information on recording a patient/client history can be found in Chapter 8.

After obtaining the patient history, the physical therapist collects objective data through (1) a systems review and (2) specific tests and measures. During the systems review, the physical therapist assesses the patient's overall condition through a gross screening of the different body systems. The gross screening includes a review of the cardiovascular and pulmonary (eg, heart rate, blood pressure, respiratory rate, and presence of edema), integumentary (eg, skin texture or pliability, scar assessment, color, and integrity), musculoskeletal (eg, symmetry, gross range of motion, gross strength, height, and weight), and neuromuscular (eg, balance, coordination, and gait) systems.[4] The physical therapist also screens the patient's cognitive and communication abilities, affect, language, and learning style(s). Additional examples for screening the various body systems can be found in defensible documentation.[4] Data collected during the history and systems review help form the basis for the tests and measures portion of the examination.

The physical therapist should use his or her clinical decision-making skills to interpret data gathered during the history and systems review to determine the most appropriate tests and measures needed. For example, a patient complaining of difficulty walking long distances may require a specific test of endurance, and a patient who demonstrates decreased lower extremity range of motion during the systems review should have specific goniometric measurements. Screening results that show an unimpaired body system should also be documented so that readers are aware of particular screenings that were performed. For example, if an integumentary screening is normal, the physical therapist documents the type of screening(s) performed and the results.

Specific tests and measures allow the physical therapist to accurately pinpoint and measure impairments in body structure and function, activity limitations, and participation restrictions. The results of the tests and measurements provide a baseline of the patient's status and guide the physical therapist in determining if the patient is appropriate to receive physical therapy services. Data collected from the history, systems review, and tests and measures also play an important role in determining the physical therapy diagnosis, prognosis, and intervention. The *Guide to Physical Therapist Practice* and the Guidelines for Physical Therapy Documentation of Patient/Client Management provide a list of measures included in the systems review and tests and measures portion of the examination. More information on recording objective data is provided in Chapter 8.

Diagnosis, Prognosis, and Intervention

The physical therapist uses data collected in the history, systems review, and tests and measures to arrive at the diagnosis, prognosis, and intervention plan. According to the Patient/Client Management Model, this is a thought process known as the *evaluation*.[1] A physical therapist establishes a diagnosis that is within his or her scope of practice after considering all clinical data from the history, systems review, and tests and measures. The diagnosis established

by the physical therapist is different from but a complement to the patient's medical diagnosis.[5] The medical diagnosis often relates to the anatomical tissues that are considered to be the source of the symptoms.[6] Physicians determine the medical diagnosis based on results found at the cellular, tissue, organ, or system level. A diagnosis established by the physical therapist is often based on the impact of the condition on the system (typically the movement system) and the whole-person level.[1] The diagnosis established by the physical therapist is a label determined by categorizing the patient's signs and symptoms, and it should be used to communicate these signs and symptoms and guide the physical therapy intervention.[1,7,8]

In physical therapy, the diagnostic label indicates the primary dysfunctions toward which the physical therapist directs treatment.[1] To date, there is no agreed-upon method to document the physical therapy diagnosis, and, clinically, it is done in a variety of ways. Examples include one, or a combination of, the following: (1) the use of categories or classifications reported in the literature, (2) the movement dysfunction that will be addressed, (3) a summary statement that links impairments to functional deficits that will be addressed, and (4) a detailed problem list that includes specific patient/client problems that will be addressed with the physical therapy intervention (Table 4-1). Jiandani and Mhatre[6] recommended that physical therapists use International Classification of Functioning, Disability and Health language in establishing the patient/client diagnosis. They reported potential benefits including providing the use of a common language, patient centeredness, ease of outcome measurement, the awareness of contextual factors, and the ability to compare across settings. In all instances, the diagnosis established by the physical therapist should be developed based on knowledge and skills within his or her professional scope of practice and jurisdictional regulations and documented in the patient's medical record.

Following the establishment of the diagnosis, the physical therapist determines the patient's prognosis, or the expected level of function at the end of the episode of care. *Prognosis* is defined as the predicted optimal level of improvement in function and the time needed to reach that level and may include incremental levels of improvement to be achieved throughout the episode of care.[1] The physical therapist arrives at the prognosis after considering factors such as the medical diagnosis; the diagnosis established by the physical therapist; contextual factors including comorbidities and complicating factors; best available evidence; the patient's expectations and goals; clinician experience with injury, disease, illness, or dysfunction; and the patient's prior level of function. The prognosis is documented by listing the expected outcome goals with an expected time frame for achievement along with an accompanying narrative that includes reasons why progress may be slower or faster than what is typically expected.

The next step in patient/client management is to determine the intervention plan. Interventions fall into

TABLE 4-1
APPROACHES TO DOCUMENTING PHYSICAL THERAPY DIAGNOSES
Document using categories or classifications reported in the literature.
Document the movement dysfunction or disorder that will be addressed.
Provide a summary statement that links impairment to function including activity limitations and/or participation restrictions.
Create a problem list that includes specific patient/client problems that will be addressed with the physical therapy intervention.

9 categories including patient/client instruction; airway clearance techniques; assistive technology; biophysical agents; functional training in self-care and domestic, work, community, social, and civic life; integumentary repair and protection techniques; manual therapy techniques; motor function training; and therapeutic exercise.[1] The physical therapist determines medically necessary interventions based on patient data, the patient's values and expectations, available resources, the setting, and the best available evidence. Interventions should be aimed at specific problems identified in the diagnosis established by the physical therapist. In the clinical documentation, the physical therapist should provide the specific intervention and skills that will be provided, the reason(s) the intervention(s) are medically necessary, and the prescription (eg, frequency and duration).

The plan of care is the culmination of the examination, diagnostic, and prognostic processes and is established in collaboration with the patient/client and those involved in his or her care.[1] The contents included in the plan of care documentation will vary between settings, but in general the contents include (1) a brief summary of the patient/client (eg, age, sex, and medical diagnosis), (2) the diagnosis established by the physical therapist, (3) the prognosis (goals, time frame, and any supporting narrative describing significant contextual factors), (4) the medically necessary skilled interventions to be provided, and (5) the therapy prescription. The prescription includes the frequency (the number of days per week) and duration (the total length of the episode of care) of services to be provided (Figure 4-1). In inpatient rehabilitation facilities, the plan of care should also include the intensity (hours per day), the estimated length of stay, and the anticipated discharge destination.[9] Physical therapists working in an acute care setting may also be required to include recommendations for discharge destination. The creation of the plan of care is the responsibility of the physical therapist, but the physical therapist

assistant uses the plan of care when seeing a patient/client for the first time and when making decisions about progression (Example 4-1).

DOCUMENTING INTERIM VISITS

Interim visits or encounters follow the initial visit and allow the physical therapist to carry out the plan of care. There are 3 types of interim documentation: treatment or daily notes, progress notes, and re-examinations/re-evaluations. The most basic interim note is the treatment note, or daily note. These are not required in all settings. In the outpatient setting, CMS has defined treatment notes as notes that serve as records of skilled intervention(s) provided and records of time taken to provide the interventions in order to justify billing codes being used.[2] They are not required to provide evidence of medical necessity or ongoing services.[2] At minimum, the treatment notes include the following: the date the service was provided, the specific intervention/modality provided and billed in language that can be compared with the claim for verification, the total timed code treatment minutes, the total treatment time in minutes (excluding time not billable), the signature and professional designation of the qualified provider who furnished or supervised the treatment (in accordance with state practice acts), and any individual who contributed to that treatment.[2] More information on timed treatment codes is provided in Chapter 12. It is important to recognize and remember that each treatment note requires documentation of the unique skills provided during the encounter and should go beyond listed exercises on a flow sheet because these do not always demonstrate the unique skills provided in the physical therapy encounter. Different facilities will have additional requirements for treatment notes. For example, an outpatient clinic may require documentation of objective data on each visit or within a specific time frame (eg, weekly).

The second type of interim documentation is a progress note. A progress note follows a reassessment of the patient's status. In a reassessment, data collection should be comprehensive and include information from the patient/client or family/caregiver regarding progress and from formal tests and measures. Data gathered should be similar to that collected on the initial visit and help the physical therapist in determining patient/client progress and the status toward the established goals. Physical therapists use reassessments to determine if the intervention is still medically necessary and to justify ongoing services.

Like with treatment notes, CMS provides specific criteria for progress notes written in an outpatient setting. The regulations state, "The progress report provides justification for the medical necessity of treatment."[2(p186)] Content requirements for progress reports include the following[2(pp185-187)]:

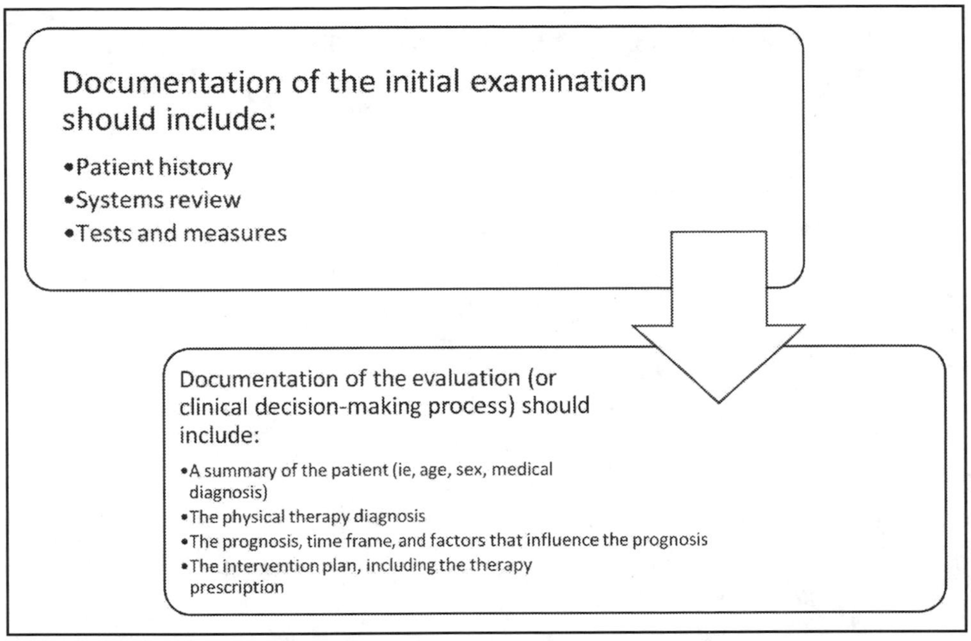

Documentation of the initial examination should include:

- Patient history
- Systems review
- Tests and measures

Documentation of the evaluation (or clinical decision-making process) should include:

- A summary of the patient (ie, age, sex, medical diagnosis)
- The physical therapy diagnosis
- The prognosis, time frame, and factors that influence the prognosis
- The intervention plan, including the therapy prescription

Figure 4-1. Overview of documentation from the initial visit.

Example 4-1. Initial Patient Documentation

Pt. name: Becky Smith

Date of service: August 1, 2019

Date of injury: July 4, 2019; 10:00 AM

Referral: Referred to physical therapist for "shoulder and elbow PROM, sling on at all other times" by Dr. John Smith

History: 62-year-old white, right-hand dominant woman, 4 weeks s/p fall from chair while changing light bulb when she sustained a (R) spiral humerus fracture. Immediately underwent ORIF and was placed in a sling. Saw the physician yesterday and was referred to physical therapy. She returns to the physician in 2 weeks. She is hoping to have the sling discontinued at that time. PMH is unremarkable. Pt. is a nonsmoker and reports being in good health. She had a hysterectomy 15 years ago.

C/C: Pain 6/10 with motion of the (R) arm movements and difficulty performing self-care skills because of decreased ability to use her (R) arm. Reports using over-the-counter ibuprofen for pain.

L/S: Pt. lives in 2-story home with her husband. She has 2 grown children living nearby who can provide assistance. She is a retired teacher who substitute teaches occasionally. Before the injury, she states that she was very active, including playing recreational tennis and walking daily. She has been unable to perform normal ADLs, including self-care, home management, driving, or exercising since the injury.

Self-report questionnaires: DASH questionnaire score 84/100; requires assistance with ADLs, including hygiene, dressing, and bathing; unable to complete home-management tasks, drive, work, or participate in normal recreational activities (eg, tennis, walking program).

Pt.'s goal: Return to her normal active lifestyle.

Systems review: Cardiopulmonary system: HR: 88, BP 128/88, RR 10; no edema. Musculoskeletal system: Pt. is 5 feet 7 inches and 155 lbs. ROM screening revealed impaired (R) UE ROM, see below. Neuromuscular system: Gross sensation to light touch in (B) UEs is intact. She ambulated into the clinic without difficulty. Integumentary system: Impaired, see below. Communication/cognition: Alert and oriented x 4. Able to communicate needs without difficulty.

Tests and measures: Capillary refill: Both hands: Intact. Integumentary integrity: Immature, 4-inch pink adhered scar present along posterior humerus, dry, hypersensitive to touch, raised ~ 1 to 2 mm. Strength: (L) UE 5/5; (R) UE N/A this visit because of surgery. PROM: (R) shoulder: flexion 96° abduction 90° ER 35° IR 50°; elbow: –10/100°. AROM: cervical WNL; (R) wrist and hand WNL; (L) shoulder: flexion 160° abduction 160° ER 90° IR 70°; elbow 0/140°.

Diagnosis, prognosis, and plan: 62-year-old right-hand dominant woman 4 weeks s/p ORIF (R) humerus referred for shoulder and elbow PROM to dominant extremity; she presents with impaired ROM and

(continued)

Example 4-1. Initial Patient Documentation (continued)

strength that have significantly limited her ability to perform (I) self-care, reaching, home tasks, work activities, recreational activities, and driving.

Problems to be addressed: Impairments: (1) decreased ROM (R) UE; (2) decreased strength (R) UE; (3) adhered scar; (4) pain 6/10. Activity limitations and participation restrictions: (1) requires assistance with ADLs; (2) unable to perform normal life roles including reaching, home management tasks, driving, work activities, and recreational activities.

Prognosis: Pt. has good social support and is motivated, demonstrating good potential to return to normal lifestyle and to meet established goals. No complicating factors identified at this time.

Discharge goals: (in 8 weeks, the patient will demonstrate):

1. AROM (R) UE 90% to 100% of (L) to allow pt. to perform ADLs, reaching, driving, work, and recreational activities
2. Strength (R) UE 4 to 4+/5 to allow return to full participation in ADLs, reaching, driving, work, and recreational activities
3. Nonadhered, mobile, painless scar
4. Pain 0/10 to allow her to return to her prior level of function

5. DASH score < 25%
6. Independence in all ADLs
7. Independence in home management
8. Driving without limitations
9. Working without limitations
10. Light recreational activities in 8 weeks with anticipated full return in 12 weeks

Interventions: Skilled services needed for mobilizing (R) shoulder and elbow while protecting healing fracture, providing education on proper hygiene/self-care while wearing the sling, and appropriately progressing activity for injury protection. She will be treated on outpatient basis 2 to 3 times per week for 8 weeks using therapeutic exercises to restore ROM and normalize soft tissue length, modalities to decrease pain, and soft tissue mobilization for scar adherence. The pt. will be progressed to more aggressive activities as able and when cleared by referring physician in order to restore function and strength. She will be provided with a home exercise program.

The pt. is in agreement with this plan.

Jane Smith, PT

- Date of the beginning and end of the reporting period that the report refers to
- Date the report was written (does not have to be within the reporting period)
- Signature and professional designation and, in the case of dictated documentation, the identification of the qualified professional who wrote the report and the date on which it was dictated
- Objective reports of the patient's relevant subjective statements
- Objective measurements (preferred) or a description of changes in status relative to each goal currently being addressed in treatment if they occur
- Any consistent method of identifying the goals may be used. Preferably, the long-term goals may be numbered (1, 2, 3, etc), and the corresponding short-term goals may be numbered and lettered (1-A, 1-B, 2-A, 2-B, etc). Identifiers on goals in the plan of care may not be changed during the episode of care to which the plan refers. New goals may be added as appropriate with new identifiers or letters. One should omit reference to a goal after it has been reported as met and signed, verifying the change

- Assessment of improvement and the extent of progress (or lack thereof) toward each goal
- Plans for continuing treatment, reference to additional evaluation results, and/or treatment plan revisions should be documented in the clinician's progress report
- Changes to long- or short-term goals, discharge, or an updated plan of care that is sent to the physician or nonphysician provider for certification of the next intervention of treatment

The timing of progress notes may depend on several factors including the patient's progress, setting, payer, and facility policy. For example, inpatient rehabilitation facilities may require weekly progress notes that correspond to interdisciplinary team meetings where the patient's progress toward goals is reviewed with other providers. Outpatient facilities usually require progress notes every 30 days for commercial insurance or every 10 visits for Medicare beneficiaries. Progress notes may not be required in acute care facilities because of the shortened length of stays. Also, patients progressing faster or slower than what was originally expected may warrant a progress note.

The third type of interim note is a re-evaluation. A re-evaluation is more formal than a reassessment accompanied by a progress note. Re-evaluations occur when there are significant changes in the patient's status. For example, a physical therapist is seeing a patient in his or her home and the patient becomes ill, requiring hospitalization. When the patient returns home and the physical therapist resumes treatment, a re-evaluation may be warranted. Re-evaluation is a separately billable service, and there are well-established guidelines as to how frequently they are allowed. The state's practice act or third-party payer guidelines often dictate how frequently a re-evaluation can be billed.

DOCUMENTING DISCHARGE

The final note in the patient/client record at the end of the episode of care is the discharge note, or summary. When the patient/client is being discharged from physical therapy, the physical therapist performs a discharge assessment and records the data in a discharge note, or summary. This note serves as a record of the patient's final subjective and objective status. It also provides a comparison of the baseline and final data and summarizes the progress toward goals. The discharge note also provides the final, or discharge, plan(s) (eg, transfer to another setting or return to work). The physical therapist should also describe how the intervention(s) helped in bringing about patient/client change. Clinicians should consider the discharge note the last opportunity to justify the medical necessity of the entire treatment in the event the record is audited.[2(p189)]

REVIEW QUESTIONS

1. Differentiate *examination* from *evaluation* as defined by the Patient/Client Management Model.
2. From whom does the history portion of the examination come?
3. List 5 questions that should be asked as part of a patient/client history.
4. The patient/client history and systems review should help guide the physical therapist in determining specific _____ to perform.
5. During the examination, the physical therapist should identify impairments in body _____ , activity _____ , participation _____ , and _____ factors.
6. The _____ is the thought process that allows the physical therapist to develop the diagnosis, prognosis, and interventions.
7. Differentiate between a treatment note and a progress note.
8. Differentiate between a regular reassessment and a re-examination/re-evaluation.
9. Physical therapists often assign a label to a patient's movement dysfunction that is different from the medical diagnosis. Describe 3 ways the physical therapist can document this established diagnosis in the medical record.
10. What is the role of the discharge note, or summary?

APPLICATION EXERCISES

Look at the following initial patient/client documentation and answer the questions:
1. Give 3 examples of impairments identified during the screening that resulted in further testing and measurements.
2. Give 3 examples of objective data that demonstrated an impairment in body structure or function.
3. Give 3 examples of data that demonstrated an activity limitation or participation restriction.
4. How did the physical therapist document his diagnosis in a manner that was different from the medical diagnosis?
5. How did this physical therapist document the contextual factors that may interfere with the plan of care?

This patient was admitted to an inpatient rehabilitation unit 4 days after transtibial amputation.

Patient Name: Robert Houston
Date: January 15, 2019
Problem: 72 y.o. male s/p (R) standard transtibial amputation 1/11/19. Referred for inpatient rehabilitation stay and treatment following amputation.
Patient history: Long history of chronic wounds on the (R) foot with recent development of osteomyelitis and gangrene; underwent transtibial amputation 1/11/19. Reports having 2 toes on his (R) foot amputated 1 year ago. PMH includes NIDDM, COPD, PVD, and HTN.
Chief complaints: Phantom pain from the right foot that can get up to 8/10, unable to walk by himself, and decreased endurance.
Medications: Current meds include Glucophage, albuterol, salmeterol, and atenolol.
Living situation: He lives alone in single-level house, with 2 steps at the entrance and no handrail.
Prior level of function: Patient is a retired carpenter. States he has never used an assistive device. Has been independent with all ADLs and IADLs prior to admission. Reports that he drove and enjoyed outdoor hobbies like fishing.
General health: Reports being in fair general health other than his leg.
Family history: Heart disease and high cholesterol.
Social history: He has one son living about 2 hours away who can assist on the weekends.

Health habits: Pt. is a nonsmoker and nondrinker, although smoked 1 pack per day for 30 years. Quit when he was 50 y.o.

Patient goals: Return to independent living, active lifestyle, including driving. Obtain a prosthetic device.

Systems review: CP system: HR 92 bpm, BP 135/88, RR 12, edema in residual limb. See below. Integumentary system: Sutures present along anterior aspect of the distal tibia; discoloration. See below. Musculoskeletal system: Impaired ROM and strength. See below. Neuromuscular system: Impaired sensation and mobility. See below. Communication/cognition: Pt. is alert and oriented ×4.

Tests and measures: Aerobic capacity: 2-minute walk test 50' (15 m); rate of perceived exertion during mobility exam was 13.

Anthropometric measurements: Residual limb length is 7" from medial knee joint line.

Girth	Right	Left
Knee joint	52 cm	50 cm
2" below	52.5 cm	48 cm

Balance: Berg Balance Score = 42; Activities-Specific Balance Scale = 40%

Posture: Forward head and rounded shoulders during sitting and standing; (L) LE under COG; (L) medial longitudinal arch flattened (pes planus)

Circulation: Capillary refill in (L) great toe time > 2 seconds

Pain assessment: NPRS best 3/10, worst 8/10; Pain Interference Scale: 41/70; location: phantom limb pain and incisional; type: burning, sharp

Peripheral nerve integrity: (L) foot sensation is intact to light touch and patient is able to sense the 10 g monofilament; decreased sensation to light touch around the scar on residual limb

Integumentary integrity: Distal residual limb 6-inch horizontal incision, minimal red bloody drainage, no tension on wound, complete closure, sutures intact, no s/s of infection; mild erythema around the incision

AROM: (R) hip flexion 100 degrees, extension 0 degrees, abduction 40 degrees, adduction 10 degrees, knee 10/60 degrees; (L) hip flexion 120 degrees, extension 0 degrees, abduction 40 degrees, adduction 10 degrees, knee flexion 0/140 degrees. (B) UEs are WNL.

PROM: Right hip flexion 120 degrees, knee 5/65 degrees capsular end feel in knee extension; soft end feel in hip flexion.

Strength: UEs 5/5; (L) LE hip 4/5, knee 4/5, ankle 4/5; (R) LE hip 4–/5, knee not tested

Mobility: w/c mobility: 20' Indpt but distance limited due to fatigue (max assist required for parts management); bed mobility: Indpt; transfers: bed to/from chair CGA ×1 with verbal cues; ambulation: 50 × 2 with min @ ×1 for balance and sequencing steps with standard walker placement

Intervention: 15 minutes of instruction in therapeutic exercises to (1) increase AROM of the (R) LE including hip flexion, extension, abduction, and adduction; knee flexion and extension (20 reps each); (2) to increase muscle function in the (R) residual limb including quad sets × 20 reps; and (3) to increase flexibility of the (R) hamstrings through towel propping

Diagnosis, prognosis, and plan:

72 y.o. male 4 days s/p transtibial amputation. Patient presents with decreased ROM, strength, endurance, and balance resulting in impaired mobility, ability to live alone, and participate in the community. Patient lives alone and will need to be safe in his home environment, also will need to take care of the sound limb during ambulation tasks due to circulation and foot posture. PMH and poor endurance may slow progress.

Impaired body structure/function:

1. Decreased ROM (R) LE
2. Decreased strength (R) LE
3. Decreased sensation (L) LE
4. Edema
5. Incision present
6. Impaired balance with walker
7. Pain, including phantom pain and interference
8. Impaired endurance

Activity limitations and participation restrictions:

1. Decreased independence with transfers
2. Decreased independence with ambulation
3. Unable to perform home management tasks
4. Unable to drive
5. Unable to perform necessary IADLs (grocery shopping, going to bank, etc)

Discharge goals: After 3 weeks, the patient will

1. Demonstrate full A/PROM in the right LE with no contractures—necessary for normal prosthetic ambulation
2. Demonstrate right LE strength 4/5 also to allow normal prosthetic ambulation
3. Be independent with skin care and monitoring skin on the residual limb and (L) LE
4. Decrease and stabilize edema to be < 1/4 inch from sound side to prepare for prosthesis.
5. Berg Balance Score > 45
6. Pain level decreased to < 3/10 at worst
7. Pain interference decreased to < 20
8. 2-minute walk test = 50 m
9. Ambulate 200' with least restrictive assistive device to allow independence with home ambulation
10. Transfer in/out of bed and sit to/from stand independently

Plan: Patient to receive services for improving ROM, strength, endurance, and balance to improve functional mobility and safety within the home environment. He will require education on use of assistive device, sound limb care, skin care, and preparing residual limb for prosthesis.

See patient for 1 hour bid for ~ 3 weeks for intensive rehabilitation to work on achieving the above goals. Patient will likely require home health upon discharge and will require consultation with prosthetist. He is motivated and agrees with the above plan.

REFERENCES

1. American Physical Therapy Association. *Guide to Physical Therapist Practice 3.0*. http://guidetoptpractice.apta.org/content/1/SEC2.body. Accessed March 29, 2019.
2. Centers for Medicare and Medicaid Services. Medicare Benefit Policy Manual. Publication no. 100-02. Chapter 15. https://www.cms.gov/Regulations-and-Guidance/Guidance/Manuals/Downloads/bp102c15.pdf. Published July 12, 2019. Accessed February 18, 2020.
3. American Physical Therapy Association. Guidelines: physical therapy documentation of patient/client management. BOD G03-05-16-41. https://www.apta.org/uploadedFiles/APTAorg/About_Us/Policies/BOD/Practice/DocumentationPatientClientMgmt.pdf. Accessed February 18, 2020
4. American Physical Therapy Association. Defensible documentation. http://www.apta.org/DefensibleDocumentation/Elements/InitialExamEval/#Examination. Published 2018. Accessed July 4, 2019.
5. Rose SJ. Musing on diagnosis (editorial). *Phys Ther*. 1988;68:1665.
6. Jiandani MP, Mhatre BS. Physical therapy diagnosis: how is it different. *J Postgrad Med*. 2018;64(2):69-72.
7. Rose SJ. Physical therapy diagnosis: role and function. *Phys Ther*. 1989;69(7):535-537.
8. Sahrmann SA. Diagnosis by the physical therapist: a prerequisite for treatment. *Phys Ther*. 1988;68:1703-1706.
9. Centers for Medicare and Medicaid Services. Medicare Benefit Policy Manual. Publication no. 100-02. Chapter 1. https://www.cms.gov/Regulations-and-Guidance/Guidance/Manuals/Downloads/bp102c01.pdf. Published March 10, 2017. Accessed February 18, 2020.

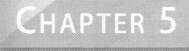

Documentation Formats

Mia L. Erickson, PT, EdD

CHAPTER OUTLINE

- Documentation Formats
  - Narrative Notes
  - Problem-Oriented Medical Record
  - Subjective, Objective, Assessment, and Plan Notes
  - Functional Outcomes Reporting
- Contemporary Practice
- Dictation
- Templates and Fill-In Forms

CHAPTER OBJECTIVES

Upon completion of this chapter, the reader will be able to:

1. Compare and contrast narrative notes, problem-oriented medical records, SOAP notes, and functional outcomes reports
2. Describe the problem-status-plan documentation format
3. Differentiate between information found in the S, O, A, and P portions of a SOAP note
4. Explain the rationale for blending functional information into SOAP
5. Organize patient information using the different documentation formats

Erickson ML, Utzman RR, McKnight RS.
Physical Therapy Documentation: From Examination to Outcome,
Third Edition (pp 33-52).
© 2020 Taylor & Francis Group.

KEY TERMS

functional outcomes report
narrative notes
problem-oriented medical record
SOAP note

KEY ABBREVIATIONS

FOR
Imp:
POMR
Pr:
SOAP
Tx:

DOCUMENTATION FORMATS

Documentation in physical therapy practice can take on a variety of formats, and the format you use will depend on the type of patients being treated, the practice setting, state laws, practice acts, reimbursement requirements, and the type of patient encounter. It will also depend on whether you are using paper-based documentation or an electronic medical record. Traditional documentation formats include narrative reports; problem-oriented medical records (POMRs), Subjective, Objective, Assessment, and Plan (SOAP) notes, functional outcomes reports (FORs), and a hybrid approach, which includes a combination of the formats mentioned. The purpose of this chapter is to discuss different formats and the positive and negative aspects of each format and to provide some examples.

Narrative Notes

In narrative documentation, the clinician describes the patient encounter with pertinent information provided in paragraph format. The narrative format can be used when documenting initial patient encounters (Example 5-1A), interim notes (Example 5-1B), re-evaluations (Example 5-1C), and discharge summaries (Example 5-1D). Besides typical patient care documentation, there are other times when the narrative format is the most appropriate to use. Narrative notes are sometimes the easiest to use when you need to describe the details of a situation or encounter and you are trying to paint a vivid description of what happened. Examples include describing a sequence of events, brief interactions with patients, conversations with other health care providers, or any other situation that requires a detailed explanation and no other documentation formats are appropriate (Example 5-1E).

Authors have identified several problems with the narrative record. First, the lack of structure combined with a high degree of variability among clinicians' writing styles make narrative notes difficult to read. It is also difficult for someone reading the note to find important information about the patient.[1] For example, it would be very time consuming for a case manager to sort through a chart filled with unstructured narrative entries to locate information regarding the patient's ability to transfer. Following the clinician's problem-solving process can also be difficult in narrative reports.[2] Because of the lack of structure, there is potential for the writer to omit important details. This can be a problem because it is assumed that if it is not documented, it did not happen. Quinn and Gordon[1] recommended that clinicians should develop an outline, or template, of necessary information to include so that important details about the encounter are not inadvertently omitted. One may also use headings to denote different sections or different types of data. Headings give the narrative note structure, making it more readable and allowing someone to find information in the note more quickly. Headings often used are shown in Table 5-1. The electronic medical record builds in headings, making the note more readable.

Problem-Oriented Medical Record

Lawrence Weed[2] developed the POMR in the 1960s. It was developed to better allow students to define patient problems, provide data to support the problems, and convey the solutions for the problems.[3] The POMR provided structure to the medical record by organizing information and treatment according to the patient's problems. The first page of the medical record included the patient's problem list, and this served as the "table of contents" for the remainder of the medical record (Example 5-2A). Subsequent entries, or interim notes, included subjective and objective clinical data, an overall impression (Imp:), treatment (Tx:) or therapy, and a future plan for each problem (Example 5-2B).

Major advantages of the POMR have been reported.[4-8] It provided organization and structure to the medical record and included a comprehensive list of the patient's problems. It allowed the reader to quickly identify care provided and future management plans for each problem. The POMR also allowed a clinician interested in a particular problem to go directly to that aspect of the note, thus easing communication among care providers. Finally, the POMR provided a chronological sequence of interventions for a particular problem, better outlining the problem-solving process.

Echternach[9] described the use of the POMR in physical therapy. He described the benefits of using this structure with physical therapist students, which included allowing students to focus on patient problems, collect objective

Example 5-1A. Initial Documentation: Narrative Format

Physical Therapy
Initial Examination and Plan of Care

Pt. name: John Smith
Date of Service: January 3, 2020
Reason for Referral: Evaluate and treat for (L) elbow pain
Physician: Dr. Jones
Chart Number: 346254

Mr. Smith is a 35-year-old left-hand dominant male with (L) elbow pain. Pt. reports developing pain after spending the weekend painting his house 3 months ago. The pt. reports using ice and taking meds (over-the-counter ibuprofen) initially, but this didn't help. Saw his physician for a yearly physical and mentioned the elbow pain. His physician suggested "trying a few weeks of PT." Chief complaint at this time is pain (6/10 at worst and 2/10 at best) that increases with heavy grip, computer use, and using hand tools. Denies temperature changes and numbness. Has not had any imaging studies. Pt. denies history of a similar problem or prior elbow pain. Reports overall health is good with no relevant medical or surgical history. Pt. lives alone and works as an accountant. Reports primary functional deficits include painful work-related activities, home-management tasks, and recreational activities, such as mountain biking and kayaking. Global functional rating is 85/100. The pt.'s goals for therapy include pain reduction allowing him to participate in functional and recreational tasks and prevention of recurrence. DASH functional assessment score 28/100. Review of systems revealed BP: 120/84, HR: 78 bpm, and RR: 12; no edema in (R) or (L) UE. Impairments noted in musculoskeletal system, see below. Neurologic screening indicated neurovascular structures are intact and sensation is WNL bil. Integumentary system screening showed normal skin color and texture. Pt. is alert and oriented x 4. There is palpable point tenderness on the (L) lateral epicondyle and wrist extensor origin. AROM of (R) UE is WNL (elbow 0/145°); (L) shoulder, forearm, wrist, and hand are WNL; (L) elbow is -10/140° with c/o pain at end range elbow flexion, extension, forearm supination, and wrist extension; cervical A/PROM also WNL and pain free. PROM of the (L) elbow is 0/145 with normal end feel but c/o pain. MMT indicates 5/5 strength throughout (B) UE except (L) wrist extension and supination are 4/5 with pain;

(+) tennis elbow test. Pain-free grip strength (R) 100, 110, 108# (L) 65, 60, 55#. Treatment today consisted of (1) self-care: instruction in HEP, activity modification including grip and activities to avoid, instruction in safe use of tennis elbow strap x 10 minutes; (2) 3 MHz US at 100% duty cycle x 4 minutes with the intensity at 1.25 W/cm^2 to (L) lateral epicondyle; (3) wrist extensor stretching with neutral and UD wrist, cross friction massage to extensor origin x 5 minutes. Total exam time 30 minutes and total tx time 19 minutes. 35-year-old left-hand dominant male with medical dx of (L) lateral elbow tendinopathy (3-month history). Pain and decreased ROM are limiting the pt.'s ability to perform functional grip and complete necessary home, work, and recreational activities. Problem list: elbow pain and tenderness; decreased AROM (L) elbow; (L) wrist and elbow weakness; decreased grip strength; painful work-related, home-management, and recreational tasks; limited in carrying heavy objects and opening/closing jars. Pt. has good potential for improvement but may require extended time due to chronic nature of his condition. Expected LTGs to be met by 3/3/20: (A) decrease pain 90% to 100% to allow normal functional tasks; (B) A/PROM (L) elbow WNL and pain free to allow normal ADLs, (C) 5/5 strength (L) UE without pain, (D) pain-free grip strength = to the (R) UE; (E) pain-free work-related, home-management, and recreational tasks; (F) no difficulty in carrying heavy objects or opening/closing jars; and (G) DASH score decreased < 10%. STGs to be met in 2 weeks: (A-1) decrease pain 10% to 20%; (B-1) increase A/PROM by 5° for flexion and extension; (C-1) strength 4+/5; (D-1) increase pain-free grip strength 10 to 15#; (E-1) decrease pain during work-related, home-management, and recreational tasks by 50%; (F-1) mild difficulty (per DASH) in carrying heavy objects or opening/closing jars; and (G-1) DASH score decreased 10% to 15%. Skilled services needed to administer modalities and friction massage to soften adhesions associated with chronic inflammation and decrease pain, teach pt. safe stretching program to increase flexibility and eccentric strengthening for appropriate connective tissue elongation, and instruct in activity modification. Physical therapy intervention will be provided 2 times per week for 6 weeks. This pt. is in agreement with the plan of care.

Sue Smith, DPT

Example 5-1B. Interim Note: Narrative Format

Physical Therapist's Interim Note

Pt. name: John Smith
Date of Service: January 6, 2020
Reason for Referral: Evaluate and treat for (L) elbow pain
Physician: Dr. Jones
Chart Number: 346254

Pt. reports pain at level 6/10 at worst and 0 to 1/10 at best. Pain still increases with heavy grip, computer use, and using hand tools. Reports compliance with HEP. No adverse effects from last tx. Palpable point tenderness on (L) lateral epicondyle and wrist extensor origin. AROM of (L) elbow is -10/140°. Treatment today consisted of (1) 3 MHz US at 100% duty cycle x 4 minutes with the intensity at 1.25 W/cm^2 to (L) lateral epicondyle; (2) wrist extensor stretching with neutral and UD wrist, cross friction massage to extensor origin x 10 minutes; (3) reviewed pt.'s HEP x 5 minutes; and (4) ice massage x 5 minutes to (L) extensor origin (total tx time = 24 minutes). Pt. notes slight improvement in pain since last visit. No other changes in objective or subjective data. Assess scapular strength next visit. Continue with current plan of care.

Sue Smith, DPT

Example 5-1C. Reassessment: Narrative Format

Physical Therapist's Reassessment and Progress Report

Pt. name: John Smith
Date of Service: January 30, 2020
Reason for Referral: Evaluate and treat for (L) elbow pain
Physician: Dr. Jones
Chart Number: 346254

Pt. has been receiving physical therapy since 1/3/20 for (L) lateral elbow tendinopathy. Chief complaint at this time is still pain (3/10 at worst and 0/10 at best). It continues to increase with heavy grip and using hand tools. No longer having pain during work-related activities. Reporting primary functional deficits at this time include painful home-management tasks and recreational activities. Global functional rating is 90/100. DASH functional assessment score 13/100. The pt.'s present therapy goals include returning to prior level of activity without pain and regaining all ROM. Musculoskeletal system shows palpable point tenderness on the (L) lateral epicondyle and wrist extensor origin. AROM of (L) elbow is -5/145° with minimal to no pain at end range elbow flexion, extension, forearm supination, or wrist extension. MMT indicates (L) wrist extension and supination are 4+/5 with pain upon extension only. Continues to have (+) tennis elbow test. Pain-free grip strength (R) 100, 110, and 108#; (L) 85, 90, and 87#. Treatment today consisted of (1) wrist extensor stretching with neutral and UD wrist, cross friction massage to extensor origin, and eccentric strengthening to wrist extensors x 15 minutes and (2) parascapular muscle strengthening 3 x 10 in prone position with manual facilitation for recruitment of scapular muscles. Total re-exam time 30 minutes and tx time 30 minutes.

Pt. has made progress with his therapy program. Worst pain has decreased from 6/10 to 3/10, pain during ADLs has decreased, and global rating of function has increased 5%. DASH functional assessment has also decreased 15%, which suggests significant change. Continues to show s/s of (L) lateral elbow tendinopathy. Pain with gripping continues to limit his home-management tasks and participation in recreational activities. Specific problems include elbow pain and tenderness, decreased AROM (L) elbow, muscle weakness, decreased grip strength, painful home-management and recreational tasks, limited in carrying heavy objects, and opening/closing jars. Pt. continues to show good potential for improvement but may require extended time due to chronicity. Expected LTGs to be met by 3/3/20: (A) decrease pain 90% to 100% to allow normal functional tasks; (B) A/PROM (L) elbow WNL and pain free to allow normal ADLs; (C) 5/5 strength (L) without pain; (D) pain-free grip strength = to the (R) UE; (E) pain-free work-related, home-management, and recreational tasks; (F) no difficulty in carrying heavy objects or opening/closing jars; and (G) DASH score decreased < 10%. STGs set at initial visit have been met. For the next 2 weeks, we will continue to work

(continued)

Example 5-1C. Reassessment: Narrative Format (continued)

toward meeting the previously LTGs seeing the pt. 1 to 2 times per week for 4 weeks. Tx will include continued stretching, eccentric and scapular strengthening, joint mobilizations, modalities if needed, and progression to return to normal activities. This pt. is in agreement with the new plan of care.

Sue Smith, DPT

Example 5-1D. Discharge Summary: Narrative Format

Discharge Summary

Pt. name: John Smith
Date of Service: February 15, 2020
Reason for Referral: Evaluate and treat for (L) elbow pain
Physician: Dr. Jones
Chart Number: 346254
Dates of PT Services: January 3 through February 15, 2020 (6 visits)

Pt. has been receiving PT for (L) lateral elbow tendinopathy since 1/3/20. At present, pain is 0/10 and occasionally goes to 1 to 2/10 with heavy activities like using hand tools. No pain with normal ADLs, home-management, recreation, community, or work activities. Denies activity limitations or participation restrictions. Global functional rating is 98/100. DASH functional score 8/100 (8%). He reports that he can perform his HEP without difficulty and the "stretching has helped." Negative palpable point tenderness; AROM (L) elbow 0/145°; wrist extension and supination strength are 5/5 and pain free; (-) tennis elbow test; pain-free grip strength (R) 100, 110, 110# and (L) 98, 105, 100#. Pt. has made good progress including improving AROM, MMT, and grip strength to normal. Also has shown reduced pain (90% to 100%) and improved function during normal ADLs, home-management, work, community, and recreational activities. All LTGs have been met. Plan to d/c PT at this time to (I) HEP. Pt. will return if further problems arise.

Sue Smith, DPT

Example 5-1E. Other Narrative Examples

Inpatient Setting:

02/09/20: Went to see pt. for gait and transfer training. Pt. lying in bed and reported feeling sick. Refused physical therapy today. *Jon Smith, PT*

05/03/20: Attempted to see pt. this afternoon. Spoke with nursing prior to session, they indicated that pt. was to receive a blood transfusion and asked to withhold physical therapy today. Will attempt to see pt. in the morning if cleared. *Jon Smith, PT*

Outpatient Setting:

04/05/20: Pt. called this morning reporting that she was not improving with therapy. Stated that she planned to call her physician. Canceled appointment for today. Will call to reschedule if needed. *Jon Smith, PT*

04/05/20: Saw pt. today for follow-up visit after fabrication and fitting of (L) WHFO wrist cock-up orthosis. Remolded edge around thenar eminence and at MCP crease to allow more thumb and finger motion and decrease skin pressure at distal palmar crease. Pt. indicated improved motion with decreased pain after adjustment. Will have pt. return if needed for further orthosis adjustments. *Jon Smith, PT*

data, progress treatment, and identify needs for changes in the treatment. Additional benefits included earlier student integration into the patient's care, improved communication between the student and the clinical instructor, and better ability to evaluate student performance and decision making. Additional authors reported on the use of the POMR in rehabilitation.[4,5,8,10]

Regardless of the benefits to the structure provided with the POMR, authors have reported problems. First, it was difficult for providers to see the "whole patient" because of its organization by individual patient problems.[6] For example, in more complex cases, it was possible that a clinician working with breathing might not be

TABLE 5-1

COMMON HEADINGS USED TO ADD STRUCTURE TO DOCUMENTATION

Patient's name	Muscle tone
Medical record number	Endurance
Date of service	Balance
Reason for referral	Integumentary
History of present illness or problem	Sensation
Mechanism of injury	Functional assessment
Chief complaint(s)	Interventions provided
Medications	Mobility
Imaging procedures/lab results	Gait
Prior and current functional status	Transfers
General health	Summary
Prior or past medical history	Medical diagnosis
Pain intensity or numeric pain rating	Physical therapist's diagnosis
Lifestyle or living situation	Problem list
Screening or systems review	Rehab potential
Observation	Complicating factors
Palpation	Short-term goals
Range of motion	Long-term goals
Strength	Planned interventions

Example 5-2A. Initial Documentation: POMR Format

Physical Therapy
Initial Examination and Plan of Care

Pt. name: John Smith
Date of Service: January 3, 2020
Reason for Referral: Evaluate and treat for (L) elbow pain
Physician: Dr. Jones
Chart Number: 346254
Problem list:

1. Elbow pain and tenderness limiting functional activities
2. Decreased AROM (L) elbow limiting ADLs
3. Muscle weakness limiting home-management, work, and recreation activities
4. Decreased grip strength
5. Painful work-related, home-management, and recreational tasks

6. Limited in carrying heavy objects and opening/closing jars

Subjective: <u>Medical dx:</u> (L) lateral elbow tendinopathy; referred to physical therapist by Dr. Jones

<u>HPI:</u> 35-year-old left-hand dominant male reports developing pain after spending the weekend painting his house 3 months ago. The pt. reports using ice and taking meds (over-the-counter ibuprofen) initially, but this didn't help. Saw his physician for a yearly physical and mentioned the elbow pain. His MD suggested "trying a few weeks of PT." Reports that he has not had any or imaging procedures. Pt. denies hx of a similar problem or prior elbow pain.

<u>C/C:</u> Pain (6/10 at worst and 2/10 at best) that increases with heavy grip, computer use, and using hand tools. Denies temperature changes and numbness. Reports primary functional deficits include painful work-related activities, home-management tasks,

(continued)

Example 5-2A. Initial Documentation: POMR Format
(continued)

and recreational activities such as mountain biking and kayaking. Global functional rating is 85/100.

<u>PMH</u>: Reports overall health is good with no relevant medical or surgical history.

<u>Lifestyle</u>: Pt. lives alone and works as an accountant.

<u>Functional assessment</u>: DASH functional assessment score 28/100.

<u>Pt.'s goals</u>: Pain reduction to allow improvement in functional tasks and prevention of recurrence.

Objective: <u>Gross ROS</u>: BP: 120/84, HR: 78 bpm, and RR: 12; no edema in (R) or (L) UE. Impairments noted in musculoskeletal system, see below. Neurologic screening indicated neurovascular structures are intact and sensation is WNL bil. Integumentary system screening showed normal skin color and texture. Pt. is alert and oriented x 4.

<u>Pain</u>: Musculoskeletal system shows palpable point tenderness on the (L) lateral epicondyle and wrist extensor origin.

<u>AROM</u>: (R) UE is WNL (elbow 0/145°); (L) shoulder, forearm, wrist, and hand are WNL except elbow is -10/140 with c/o pain at end range elbow flexion, extension, forearm supination and wrist extension; cervical A/PROM also WNL and pain free.

<u>PROM</u>: (L) elbow is 0/145 with normal end feel but c/o pain.

<u>Strength</u>: MMT indicates 5/5 strength throughout (B) UE except (L) wrist extension and supination are 4/5 with pain. All special provocation tests for (L) elbow are unremarkable except a (+) tennis elbow test. Pain free grip strength (R) 100, 110, 108#; (L) 65, 60, 55#.

<u>Time</u>: Exam: 30 minutes

Imp: Pain, ROM loss, and weakness are limiting the pt.'s ability to grip, carry heavy objects, open/close lids, perform full home-management duties, and participate in normal work tasks. Physical therapist's dx: impaired mobility, function, muscle performance and ROM due to connective tissue dysfunction. Pt.

has good potential for improvement but may require extended time due to chronicity.

<u>Expected LTGs</u>: to be met by 03/03/20: (A) decrease pain 90% to 100% to improve ADLs; (B) A/PROM (L) elbow WNL and pain free to improve ADLs; (C) 5/5 strength (L) without pain to improve functional tasks; (D) pain-free grip strength = (R) to improve functional tasks; (E) pain-free work-related, home-management, and recreational tasks; (F) no difficulty in carrying heavy objects or opening/closing jars; and (G) DASH score < 10%.

<u>STGs</u>: to be met in 2 weeks: (A-1) decrease pain 10% to 20%; (B-1) increase A/PROM by 5° for flexion and extension; (C-1) strength 4+/5; (D-1) increase pain-free grip strength 10 to 15#; (E-1) decrease pain during work-related, home-management, and recreational tasks by 50%; (F-1) mild difficulty (per DASH) in carrying heavy objects or opening/closing jars; and (G-1) DASH score decreased 10% to 15%.

<u>Tx today</u>: (1) Education in self-care: HEP, activity modification to decreased tight fisting and overuse activities, discussed activities to avoid and modified handle grips; proper use of tennis elbow strap and (2) 3 MHz US at 100% duty cycle x 4 minutes with the intensity at 1.25 W/cm^2 to (L) lateral epicondyle, wrist extensor stretching with neutral and UD wrist, cross friction massage to extensor origin. Tx time: 16 minutes.

Plan: Skilled services are needed to administer modalities and friction massage to soften adhesions associated with chronic inflammation and teach pt. safe stretching program to increase flexibility, eccentric strengthening for appropriate connective tissue elongation, and activity modification. Physical therapy interventions will be provided 2 times per week for 6 weeks. This pt. is in agreement with the plan of care.

Sue Smith, DPT

aware of postural problems without reading separate chart entries and that could be incredibly time consuming. In addition, for patients with multiple problems, the POMR became increasingly complex, requiring an extraordinary amount of time for an individual who is managing multiple problems.

A more recent problem-oriented approach, although it did not evolve from the POMR, is the problem-status-plan approach. In this format, one documents the patient's functional problem, his or her current functional status, the day's intervention(s) addressing the problem, and the rehabilitative plans that will be performed (Example 5-3). Using this approach, the reader is able to identify the problem for which each intervention is directed. This approach is often used in documenting interim notes for early intervention and school-based settings, and it can be useful for parents.

Example 5-2B. Interim Note: POMR Format

Physical Therapist's Interim Note

A separate entry for each problem is completed; therefore, for this date of service, there would be potentially 6 entries in the chart. Two entries are provided as examples using this format.

Pt. name: John Smith
Date of Service: January 6, 2020
Reason for Referral: Evaluate and treat for (L) elbow pain
Physician: Dr. Jones
Chart Number: 346254
Problem List:

1. Elbow pain and tenderness limiting functional activities
2. Decreased AROM (L) elbow limiting ADLs
3. Muscle weakness limiting home-management, work, and recreation activities
4. Decreased grip strength
5. Painful work-related, home-management, and recreational tasks
6. Limited in carrying heavy objects and opening/closing jars

Note for Problem #1: Elbow pain and tenderness limiting functional activities
S: Pt. reports pain at level 6/10 at worst and 0 to 1/10 at best. Pain still increases with heavy grip, computer use, and using hand tools. Reports compliance with HEP. **O:** Palpable point tenderness on (L) lateral epicondyle and wrist extensor origin. Treatment today consisted of (1) 3 MHz US at 100% duty cycle x 4 minutes with the intensity at 1.25 W/cm^2 to (L) lateral epicondyle, (2) reviewed pt.'s HEP x 5 minutes, and (3) ice massage x 5 minutes to (L) extensor origin. (Total tx time 14 minutes).
Imp: Pt. notes slight improvement in pain since last visit as evidenced by decrease in pain. No other changes in objective or subjective data.
Plan: Continue with current plan of care.

Sue Smith, DPT

Note for Problem #2: Decreased AROM (L) elbow limiting ADLs: no subjective comments on ROM
O: AROM of (L) elbow is -10/140°. Treatment today consisted of (1) wrist extensor stretching with neutral and UD wrist, cross friction massage to extensor origin
Imp: No changes in ROM since initial visit.
Plan: Continue with current plan of care.

Sue Smith, DPT

Subjective, Objective, Assessment, and Plan Notes

The SOAP acronym stands for Subjective, Objective, Assessment, and Plan. The SOAP documentation format evolved from the POMR initially described by Weed.[2] The SOAP format provided structure to the entries that described patient problems and their management. Because of the difficulty in using the POMR when managing complex patients, clinicians began using the SOAP format as a stand-alone documentation format that contained documentation for all patient problems within a single chart entry. Nevertheless, the SOAP format is ubiquitous and is widely used by medical and rehabilitation professionals, and its components—S, O, A, and P—are well established in electronic medical record documentation.

In the SOAP note, the S, or subjective section, includes anything the patient tells you pertaining to his or her injury, disease, condition, or illness. The subjective section also includes any information provided by the patient's family or caregivers. The O, or objective, section includes the results of relevant tests and measures, the patient's functional status, and physical therapy interventions performed for that day of service. The A, or assessment, includes the interpretation, or impression, of the patient's condition in the context of all data that have been collected, and the P stands for plan. It includes any plans for managing the patient and his or her physical therapy problems. Specific information provided in the S, O, A, and P portions of the notes can be found in Figures 5-1 through 5-4. A "problem" (Pr:) section may precede the SOAP note. When used, the problem section contains information pertaining to the medical diagnosis, the physical therapy referral, and/or information from the medical record (Example 5-4A). There is more about the problem and specific SOAP contents in subsequent chapters. The SOAP note format has become ubiquitous. It is used throughout health care, and it is integrated into electronic medical record platforms. The SOAP structure can be used for the initial encounter

Example 5-3. Documentation Using the Problem-Status-Plan Approach

PROBLEM	CURRENT STATUS	INTERVENTION	PLAN
Dependent sit-to-stand transfers	Transfers sit-to-stand with mod @ x 1	15' therapeutic exercises including: bridging, mini-squats, quad strengthening	Progress LE strengthening program
Unable to ambulate independently in the home because of fall risk	Timed up and go score 13 s; ambulates 150' with cane and supervision	15' balance activities with verbal assist for upright posture and trunk support	Progress balance program with assist for safety
Unable to perform community ambulation	Uses w/c with assist from wife for community mobility	15' gait training to increase gait velocity, independence, and safety	Progress gait training as pt.'s safety increases

documentation (see Example 5-4A), interim notes (Example 5-4B), and discharge summaries (Example 5-4C).

Although the SOAP format provides a consistent documentation format and is widely used, negative aspects of the SOAP format have been reported in the literature. Historically, the subjective section has centered on the patient's complaints, primarily pain, and rarely included subjective reports of improvements in activity limitations or participation restrictions. Second, objective findings focused on documenting data related to patient impairments, such as range of motion, rather than objective reports of functional performance. If no data were collected, the objective section remained blank. Assessments were written in terms of how the patient tolerated the treatment (eg, "The patient tolerated the treatment well.") rather than how patients were progressing, and the plan was often written in very general terms (eg, documenting "Continue per plan" repeatedly). Contents of the SOAP note were often incomplete or deficient. Also, in the original SOAP format, there was nowhere to document the treatment for the day. In their original form, SOAP notes have not provided explicit relationships between subjective complaints, objective measures, and treatment. There has also been a lack of detail on how the contextual factors influence the prognosis. Additionally, the relationship between interventions and improvement has been implied rather than explained. More recent issues with the traditional SOAP format are the tendency to leave out (1) the description of the skill used by the clinician providing the services and (2) the discussion of why treatment is medically necessary. Both of these are required for more contemporary documentation.

Clinicians using SOAP as a decision-making tool could be collecting an abundance of subjective and objective data and leaving the problem solving, or hypothesis development, for later in the initial visit. This is a problem because clinicians tend to develop a hypothesis early on in the initial visit and then test and refine it throughout the data collection.

The traditional SOAP format can be an appropriate format for learning the structure of a note, but the contents of the note are the responsibility of the provider, and the contents need to be consistent with contemporary practice, including concepts such as disablement, patient function and dysfunction, medical necessity, and the need for skilled care. The SOAP note must be written so that decisions established and written in the plan of care are supported by data in the subjective and objective sections. Also, the use of the SOAP documentation structure should not hinder the clinician's hypothesis development, whether that occurs upon meeting the patient or during the patient history. The SOAP structure is merely intended to be a format for organizing information placed or written into a medical record.

Functional Outcomes Reporting

There is a need today for integrating more function into the patient's medical record. Impairment data are needed, but many payers and facilities are requiring the emphasis of documentation be on patient function and dysfunction. Using functional terminology helps improve readability for non–health care providers reviewing documentation.[1,11] Quinn and Gordon[1] described the FOR as a type of documentation that focuses on the patient's ability to perform meaningful functional activities rather than isolated impairments. In using the FOR, the writer emphasizes the relationship between the patient's impairments and his or her activity limitations and participation restrictions. Abeln[11] suggested making the following additions to SOAP in order to integrate more functional concepts:

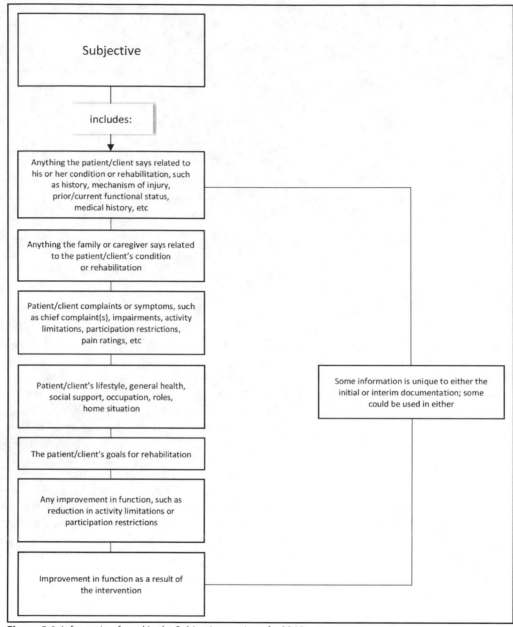

Figure 5-1. Information found in the Subjective section of a SOAP note.

1. Subjective (S) section: describe the functional problems as stated by the patient
2. Objective (O) section: assess and objectively measure the patient's functional status, including functional activities that are specific to that patient
3. Assessment (A) section:
   a. List only those impairments being addressed with therapy
   b. Describe how improvement in impairments will lead to improvement in function limitations
   c. Provide complicating factors, such as comorbidities
   d. Write goals using functional terminology

The FOR is not considered a stand-alone format, but the concepts described by these authors can easily be integrated into a documentation format.

CONTEMPORARY PRACTICE

This chapter outlines several different formats to document patient/client management. In clinical practice, you are likely to encounter a variety of documentation formats. In real-world clinical practice, you are likely to apply principles from the different formats; therefore, it is important to be familiar with each. It is the author's experience that the SOAP format is the most widely used, but the integration of

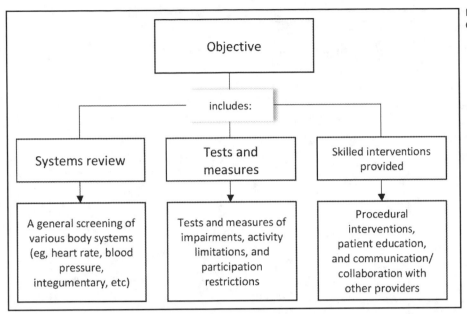

Figure 5-2. Information found in the Objective section of a SOAP note.

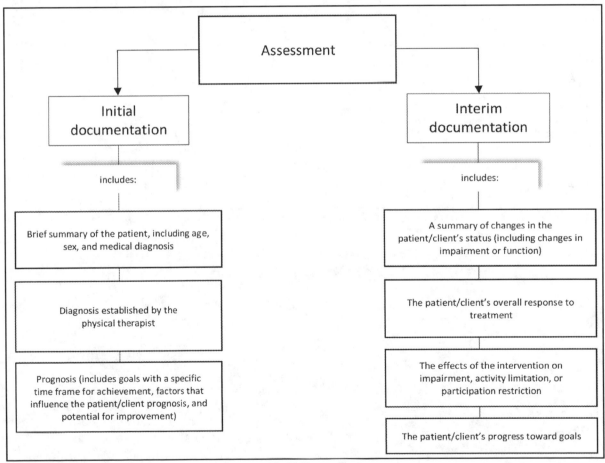

Figure 5-3. Information found in the Assessment section of a SOAP note.

patient function (like that described in the FOR) is common and required by facilities and third-party payers. At times, there will be a need to use different formats (ie, narrative). The Patient/Client Management Model also provides a framework for documentation. The examination includes the subjective and objective data, whereas the evaluation includes the diagnosis, prognosis, and plan of care. In using an electronic medical record, the format will likely be built into the software's infrastructure. Regardless, one should adhere to facility policy, and there should be some consistency in the documentation format used between patients and providers.

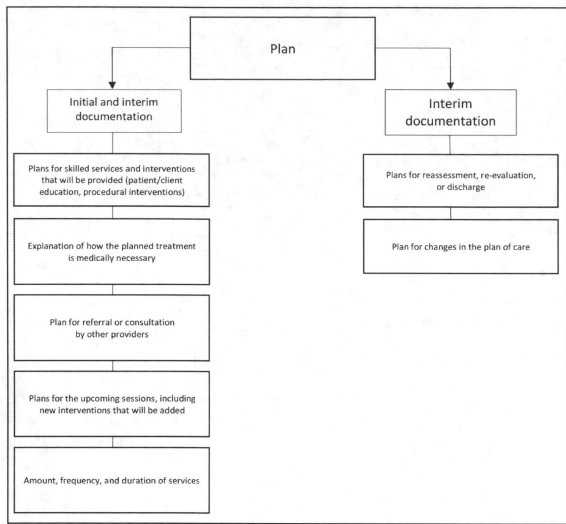

Figure 5-4. Information found in the Plan section of a SOAP note.

Example 5-4A. Initial Documentation: SOAP Format

Physical Therapy
Initial Examination and Plan of Care

Pt. name: John Smith
Date of Service: January 3, 2020
Physician: Dr. Jones
Chart Number: 346254
Pr: (L) lateral elbow tendinopathy
S: HPI: 35-year-old left-hand dominant male reports developing pain after spending the weekend painting his house 3 months ago. The pt. reports using ice and taking meds (over-the-counter ibuprofen) initially, but this didn't help. Saw his physician for a yearly physical and mentioned the elbow pain. His physician suggested "trying a few weeks of physical therapy." Has not had any imaging procedures. Pt. denies history of a similar problem and prior elbow pain.

C/C: Pain (6/10 at worst and 2/10 at best) that increases with heavy grip, computer use, using hand tools. Denies temperature changes and numbness. Reports primary functional deficits include painful work-related activities, home-management tasks, and recreational activities, such as mountain biking and kayaking. Global functional rating is 85/100.

PMH: Reports overall health is good with no relevant medical or surgical history.

L/S: Pt. lives alone and works as an accountant.

Self-report questionnaire: DASH functional assessment score 28/100.

(continued)

Example 5-4A. Initial Documentation: SOAP Format
(continued)

Pt.'s goals: Pain reduction allowing improvement in functional tasks and prevention of recurrence.

O: Gross review of systems: BP: 120/84, HR: 78 bpm, and RR: 12; no edema in (R) or (L) UE. Impairments noted in musculoskeletal system, see below. Neurologic screening indicated neurovascular structures are intact and sensation is WNL bil. Integumentary system screening showed normal skin color and texture. Pt. is alert and oriented x 4.

Pain: Musculoskeletal system shows palpable point tenderness on the (L) lateral epicondyle and wrist extensor origin.

AROM: (R) UE is WNL (elbow 0/145°); (L) shoulder, wrist, and hand are WNL except elbow is -10/140; c/o pain at end range elbow flexion, extension, forearm supination, and wrist extension; cervical A/PROM also WNL and pain free.

PROM: (L) elbow is 0/145 with normal end feel but c/o pain.

Strength: MMT indicates 5/5 strength throughout (B) UE except (L) wrist extension and supination are 4/5 with pain. All special provocation tests for (L) elbow are unremarkable except a (+) tennis elbow test. Pain-free grip strength (R) 100, 110, 108# (L) 65, 60, 55# with pain.

Tx today: (1) self-care: HEP, activity modification, use of tennis elbow strap during times of increased wrist activity x 10 minutes, (2) 3 MHz US at 100% duty cycle x 4 minutes with the intensity at 1.25 W/cm² to (L) lateral epicondyle, (3) wrist extensor stretching with neutral and UD wrist 30 seconds x 5, 4) cross friction massage to extensor origin x 3 minutes. Time: exam: 30 minutes; treatment: 21 minutes; total: 50 minutes.

A: 35-year-old left-hand dominant male with medical dx of (L) lateral elbow tendinopathy (3-month history) and physical therapist's dx: pain, impaired ROM and strength limiting ADLs, home-management, and work and recreational activities.

Problem list: elbow pain and tenderness; decreased AROM (L) elbow; (L) wrist and elbow weakness; decreased grip strength; painful work-related, home-management, and recreational tasks; limited in carrying heavy objects and opening/closing jars.

Rehab potential: Good potential for improvement but may require extended time due to chronic nature of his condition.

Expected LTGs: to be met by 3/3/20:

(A) Decrease pain 90% to 100% to allow improved function such as grip

(B) A/PROM (L) elbow WNL and pain free to improve ADLs

(C) 5/5 strength (L) without pain to improve home-management and recreational activities

(D) Pain-free grip strength equal to the (R)

(E) Pain-free work-related, home-management, and recreational tasks

(F) No difficulty in carrying heavy objects or opening/closing jars

(G) DASH score decreased to < 10%

STGs: to be met in 2 weeks

(A-1) Decrease pain 10% to 20%

(B-1) Increase A/PROM by 5° for flexion and extension

(C-1) Strength 4+/5

(D-1) Increase pain free grip strength 10 to 15#

(E-1) Decrease pain during work-related, home-management, and recreational tasks by 50%

(F-1) Mild difficulty (per DASH) in carrying heavy objects or opening/closing jars

(G-1) DASH score decreased 10% to 15%

P: Skilled services are needed to administer modalities and friction massage to soften adhesions associated with chronic inflammation and decrease pain; will also teach pt. safe stretching program to increase flexibility and eccentric strengthening for appropriate connective tissue elongation; and will instruct in activity modification. PT intervention will be provided 2 times per week for 6 weeks. This pt. is in agreement with the plan of care.

Sue Smith, DPT

The authors of this text have selected the basic SOAP format to provide a framework for learning documentation skills. This is not to suggest that clinical decision making should follow the SOAP format but rather to provide readers with some familiarity to this format due to its widespread use. For example, readers will be exposed to information that should go into the S, O, A, and P portions of the note. In addition, readers will be exposed to how aspects of the Patient/Client Management Model can fit into the basic SOAP structure (Table 5-2). The SOAP format was selected because of its prevalence in clinical practice and because of its adaptability to a variety of documentation styles and physical therapy practice settings. It is also a good format for students who are learning basic documentation skills.

Example 5-4B. Interim Note: SOAP Format

Physical Therapist's Interim Note

Pt. name: John Smith
Date of Service: January 6, 2020
Physician: Dr. Jones
Chart Number: 346254
Pr: (L) lateral elbow tendinopathy
S: Pt. reports pain at level 6/10 at worst and 0 to 1/10 at best. Pain still increases with heavy grip, computer use, and using hand tools. Reports compliance with HEP. No adverse effects from last tx.
O: Palpable point tenderness on (L) lateral epicondyle and wrist extensor origin. AROM: (L) elbow is -10/140°.

Treatment today: (1) 3 MHz US at 100% duty cycle x 4 minutes with the intensity at 1.25 W/cm^2 to (L) lateral epicondyle; (2) wrist extensor stretching with neutral and UD wrist 30 second hold x 5 reps, cross friction massage to extensor origin x 3 minutes; (3) reviewed pt.'s HEP x 5 minutes; and (4) ice massage x 5 minutes to (L) extensor origin (total tx time 20 minutes).
A: Pt. notes slight improvement in pain since last visit (0 to 1/10 from 2/10). No other changes in objective or subjective data.
P: Continue with current plan of care. Examine strength of the scapular stabilizers at the next visit.

Sue Smith, DPT

Example 5-4C. Discharge Summary: SOAP Format

Discharge Summary

Pt. name: John Smith
Date of Service: February 15, 2020
Physician: Dr. Jones
Chart Number: 346254
Dates of PT Services: January 3 through February 15, 2020 (6 visits)
Pr: (L) lateral elbow tendinopathy
S: C/C: At present pain is 0/10 and occasionally goes to 1 to 2/10 with heavy activities like using hand tools. No pain with normal ADLs, home-management, recreation, community, or work activities. Denies activity limitations or participation restrictions. Global functional rating is 98/100. He reports that he can perform his HEP without difficulty and the "stretching has helped."

O: Pain: Negative palpable point tenderness; AROM: (L) elbow 0/145°; Strength: wrist extension and supination strength are 5/5 and pain free; (-) tennis elbow test; Pain free grip strength (R) 100, 110, 110# and (L) 98, 105, 100#; Function: DASH functional score 8/100 (8%).
A: Pt. has made good progress including improving AROM, MMT, and grip strength to normal. Also has shown reduced pain (90% to 100%) and improved function during normal ADLs, home-management, work, community, and recreational activities (initial DASH score 28/100, current 8/100). LTGs: All have been met.
P: d/c physical therapy at this time to (I) HEP. Pt. will return if further problems arise.

Sue Smith, DPT

The authors believe teaching the SOAP format provides learners with the essential knowledge of required components. Once in the clinical setting, the individual can reorganize the components into the clinical setting's format, transferring what they have learned about the traditional SOAP structure into the setting's format.

Clinical decision-making models and well-written clinical documentation should not depend on or be determined by the documentation format being used; the key to quality documentation is the content. Well-written records include pertinent patient data and justify a reasonable, medically necessary, and skilled plan of care. Well-written records are necessary for physical therapy practice, and, therefore, quality and content are emphasized rather than format.

DICTATION

Dictation is verbal communication of information that is transcribed by an individual or computer software into written documentation. Transcription occurs in real time as the clinician speaks or at a later time from a recording. There is generally a format expectation (eg, the SOAP format) for transcribed records that is determined by the facility, although flexibility is allowed within that structure.

	TABLE 5-2		
RELATIONSHIP BETWEEN COMPONENTS OF THE PATIENT/CLIENT MANAGEMENT MODEL AND THEIR LOCATION IN INITIAL DOCUMENTATION USING THE SOAP FORMAT			
PATIENT/CLIENT MANAGEMENT MODEL	**INCLUDES**	**WHAT TO RECORD**	**LOCATION IN THE SOAP FORMAT**
Examination	1. History	Subjective history	Subjective (S)
	2. Systems review Cardiovascular system Integumentary system Musculoskeletal system Neuromuscular system Cognition/communication 3. Tests and measures	Objective data ○ Results of the systems review ○ Results of tests and measures	Objective (O)
Evaluation	Clinical judgment, problem-solving process, determining the physical therapy diagnosis, prognosis, and the plan of care	Brief summary of the patient including age, sex, medical diagnosis, and other pertinent information Diagnosis established by the physical therapist that includes problems that will be addressed in the physical therapy plan of care Prognosis including goals with a specific time frame for achievement, factors influencing treatment, and rehab potential	Assessment (A)
		Planned skilled interventions and rationale to give medical necessity Plans for referral to another health care provider Frequency, duration, and amount of treatment Any ultimate plans for discharge	Plan (P)
Additional Reading: American Physical Therapy Association. Defensible documentation. www.apta.org/DefensibleDocumentation. Accessed April 3, 2019.			

Dictation can be a time-saver once a clinician becomes familiar with the activity because it takes less time to speak information than to write it. An additional benefit of dictation and transcription is the documentation's readability. This leads to a reduction of error in clinical practice due to the inability to read the health care provider's handwriting. Drawbacks of dictation include the cost, hardware, typographical errors, and the error due to the transcriptionist's inability to accurately hear or understand the clinician's voice, although digital recorders are improving this area.

When dictating, it is important for the clinician to speak clearly and include any details that need to be included in the final document. In this instance, care must be taken to clearly describe how the final transcription should appear. For example, the clinician will need to verbalize if the information needs to be in a table format or when there is a new heading. Once transcription is complete, the clinician should read all transcribed notes for errors. Errors should be corrected on the original form in the same manner as all error correction for patient care documentation.

TEMPLATES AND FILL-IN FORMS

With the increasing use of the electronic medical record, paper-based templates and fill-in forms have quickly become obsolete. More often, templates and fill-in forms are built into the electronic medical record infrastructure. The use of electronic templates and forms can minimize the amount of typing required, and well-designed templates and forms can facilitate accuracy, prompt clinicians to provide necessary data, improve consistency in documentation across patients and providers, and help meet documentation guidelines set forth by third-party payers. Templates or fill-in forms can be used for initial documentation, interim notes, re-evaluations, discharge summaries, and progress letters written to physicians.

In some settings, standard templates and forms provide a mechanism for interprofessional documentation in which each discipline has its own section to complete on the same form. In some settings, federal regulations require the use of specialized forms. For example, Medicare requires the Minimum Data Set (version 3.0 was the version used at the time of writing this text) in skilled nursing facilities,[12] the Inpatient Rehabilitation Facility Patient Assessment Instrument in inpatient rehabilitation hospitals,[13] and the Outcome and Assessment Information Set in home health.[14] The Individuals with Disabilities in Education Act—a federal law that governs states to provide a free appropriate public education for all children with disabilities residing in the state between birth and age 21 years—requires therapists in early intervention and school-based programs to complete special kinds of multidisciplinary documentation.[15] Therapists working in early intervention programs (birth to age 3 years) complete documentation known as an Individualized Family Service Plan. Therapists working in a school-based setting complete an Individualized Education Plan.[15]

Clinical, or critical, pathways are another type of interprofessional documentation performed in settings where providers treat a high volume of certain patient types. These are useful when there are specific goals or expectations for each day of service following a specific surgery or procedure (eg, out of bed, transfer, ambulate, or stairs) and there are multiple service providers (eg, nursing, physical therapy, and nutrition) (Table 5-3).

A disadvantage of templates and forms is that, if not carefully designed, a form may not allow for complete documentation of all pertinent information.[20] Within any electronic system, there should be a mechanism for the clinician to include any pertinent patient information. For example, there should be a section that allows documentation of unique aspects of the treatment encounter not provided on the standard template. It is important that the therapist not be constrained by limits of a form. This is especially true for students who might feel as though they cannot deviate from the form. Additionally, templates and forms are often geared toward the patient population treated most at the facility, and it might be difficult to use these forms when documenting care provided to patients with less common diagnoses.

REVIEW QUESTIONS

1. Describe the similarities and differences between narrative notes, SOAP notes, POMRs, and FORs.
2. Give examples of information that is found in the S, O, A, and P sections of the SOAP note.
3. Why is it important to document patient status?
4. How should a patient's functional status be integrated into documentation using the SOAP format?
5. How should the International Classification of Functioning, Disability and Health and disablement concepts be integrated into the SOAP structure?
6. How should the elements of the Patient/Client Management Model be integrated into the SOAP structure?
7. What is the problem-status-plan note?
8. What are the positive and negative aspects of templates and forms?
9. What specialized documentation is required upon entrance into a skilled nursing facility? Home Health Agency? Inpatient Rehabilitation Facility?
10. At what point in the patient encounter does hypothesis development typically occur? How does using a SOAP note as a framework for hypothesis development influence this timing?

APPLICATION EXERCISES

1. Read the following statements and determine if it would belong in the S, O, A, or P section of a SOAP note.
    a. __ Gait: ambulated 50' × 2 WBAT (R) LE with min ⓐ ×1 & verbal cues to advance the (R) LE
    b. __ The patient reports the HEP has helped increase AROM
    c. __ The patient will return 2 times per week for 4 weeks
    d. __ Transfers: bed to/from chair with mod ⓐ ×2; requires stabilization to block the knee and assist to stand
    e. __ Mr. Smith is progressing toward goals set on the initial evaluation
    f. __ Patient's wife stated that she has been assisting the patient with his HEP
    g. __ Speak with the physician about decrease in BP upon transferring from supine to sitting position

TABLE 5-3

HYPOTHETICAL CLINICAL PATHWAY FOR PATIENT POST–TOTAL HIP ARTHROPLASTY

	MOBILITY (PHYSICAL THERAPY)	EXERCISE (PHYSICAL THERAPY)	SELF-CARE (OCCUPATIONAL THERAPY)	PRECAUTIONS (PHYSICAL THERAPY/ OCCUPATION THERAPY)
POSTOPERATIVE DAY 1 DATE: 7/7/19	AM treatment: Transferred supine to sit and bed to w/c with mod @ x 1 for weight bearing and safety. Sit to stand with min @ x 1. Patient ambulated in parallel bars PWB 50% with min @ x 1 for verbal instructions and safety due to light-headedness. PM treatment: Patient ambulated 20' with standard walker with min @ x 1 for verbal cueing for weight bearing precautions and safety due to light-headedness.	Patient instructed in bedside exercises bid. Performed 25 reps: 1. Ankle pumps 2. Quadriceps isometrics 3. Hip abduction 4. Heel slides 5. Gluteal isometrics		Provided patient with hip precautions; patient verbalized understanding
DAILY GOAL(S)	Out of bed to physical therapy department Ambulates 15-25' (50% weight bearing) with minimal to moderate assist x 1	Bedside exercises per protocol to increase ROM and circulation	Self-hygiene at sink with minimal assistance	Hip precautions provided
	Goal met	Goal met		Goal met
ADDITIONAL NOTE IN CHART?	Yes ✓ No ____		Yes ____ No ____	
TREATMENT TIME	28'	10'		2'
SIGNATURE	Susan Smith, PT	Susan Smith, PT		Susan Smith, PT (continued)

h. __ AROM: (R) knee 0 to 135 degrees

i. __ Improvements in knee AROM allow Mr. Smith to sit without difficulty and ascend/descend stairs with less difficulty

j. __ The patient feels that he is benefiting from the strengthening exercises in that he is now able to open jars and lids without difficulty

k. __ Mrs. Jones will be seen for gait training bid

l. __ The patient denies use of assistive device prior to admission

m. __ The patient's gait distance improved from 25' to 150' and he is now requiring supervision rather than min ⓐ ×1

n. __ The patient is demonstrating (L) neglect making her unsafe during gait and transfers

o. __ Muscle performance: all (R) LE strength is 5/5

		TABLE 5-3 (CONTINUED)		
		HYPOTHETICAL CLINICAL PATHWAY FOR PATIENT POST–TOTAL HIP ARTHROPLASTY		
	MOBILITY (PHYSICAL THERAPY)	**EXERCISE (PHYSICAL THERAPY)**	**SELF-CARE (OCCUPATIONAL THERAPY)**	**PRECAUTIONS (PHYSICAL THERAPY/ OCCUPATION THERAPY)**
POSTOPERATIVE DAY 2 **DATE:** _7/8/19_	_AM treatment: Transferred supine to sit and bed to w/c with min (a) x 1 for maintaining hip precautions and safety. Sit to stand with min (a) x 1. Patient ambulated 50' with standard walker with CGA x 1 for verbal cueing for reminders for weight-bearing precautions and sequencing gait patter_ _PM treatment: Same as AM_	_Patient instructed in bedside exercises bid. Performed 25 reps of the following:_ 1. _Ankle pumps_ 2. _Quadriceps isometrics_ 3. _Hip abduction_ 4. _Heel slides_ 5. _Gluteal isometrics_		_Patient able to verbally provide hip precautions with minimal prompts_
DAILY GOAL(S)	Out of bed to physical therapy department Ambulates 25-50' (50% weight bearing) with minimal to moderate assist x 1	Bedside exercises with cueing to increase ROM and circulation	Self-care at sink performed with verbal cues	Patient able to verbalize hip precautions
	Goal met	_Goal met_		_Goal met_
ADDITIONAL NOTE IN CHART?	Yes __✓__ No _____		Yes _____ No _____	
TREATMENT TIME	_28'_	_10'_		_2'_
SIGNATURE	_Susan Smith, PT_	_Susan Smith, PT_		_Susan Smith, PT_

Italicized text indicates aspects of the note written by the physical therapist.

p. __Vital signs:__ HR, 95 bpm; RR, 12; BP, 140/95

q. ___ The patient has improved his ability to transfer in/out of bed since initial visit and is now independent

r. ___ Will contact physician about possible d/c as patient is no longer benefiting from the intervention

s. ___ The patient's endurance is poor because of inactivity

t. ___ The patient c/o inability to brush teeth and eat with (R) hand because of decreased AROM of the (R) elbow

u. ___ The patient is unable to drive or perform safe community mobility at this time

v. ___ Edema in (R) ankle has decreased 2 cm

w. ___ __Wound appearance:__ 100% red, healthy granulation tissue with minimal drainage

2. Of the previous statements, which would be considered "functional"?

3. Of the previous statements, which integrate treatment with impairment and/or function?

4. Look at the initial documentation that follows. Answer the following questions:

   a. Which documentation format is being used: narrative, POMR, SOAP, or FOR?

   b. Identify 3 pieces of subjective data.

c. Identify 3 pieces of objective data.

d. Based on the subjective and objective data, identify the activity limitations and participation restrictions.

e. Identify the physical therapist's diagnosis.

f. How did the physical therapist describe the need for skilled care?

g. How did the physical therapist document medical necessity for services provided?

h. What information or data should the physical therapist collect and record in an interim note to show changes in status or progress from the initial session? In what section(s) would the physical therapist describe these changes?

i. What would be the most appropriate format for an interim note? Why?

Date: March 1, 2019; 11:00

Pr: 27 y.o. male s/p (L) wrist & ankle fx; referred to outpatient physical therapy to begin gentle wrist and ankle AROM and PROM and gait training with crutches using a (L) UE platform. PWB 50% (L) LE.

S: HPI: 4 wks. s/p fall (~25') from a logging truck landing on his (L) side (2/1/19). Pt. sustained fx of the (L) distal radius and ulna and (L) distal tibia & fibula. Additional injuries included 4 rib fractures on the left and a pelvic fracture. Pt. underwent ORIF for the wrist and ankle immediately after the injury. He was placed in a short-arm cast for the UE and short-leg cast for the LE. He was NWB on the (L) LE and has been unable to use crutches because he was not allowed to bear weight on the affected UE. At the time of the fall, the pt. also sustained a mild concussion. He was hospitalized for 3 days following the injury. While hospitalized, he received inpatient physical therapy to learn how to negotiate his w/c and transfer in/out bed. Both casts were removed yesterday, and his wrist was placed in a removable orthosis. Reports taking ibuprofen PRN for pain.

C/C: Pain (pain scale = 2/10) & stiffness in (L) UE & LE with decreased functional use of both. Doesn't like using w/c for mobility because it is difficult to navigate in his home. Unable to work. Requiring assist with self-care activities and home management.

Living situation: RHD; lives with wife and 2 small children in single-level home with 2 steps at entrance and handrail on the (R). Prior to injury, pt. was employed as a construction worker. He has been off work since the injury. Pt. is unable to drive and is relying on his wife and mother for transportation. No significant PMH or history of fracture. Reports being a nonsmoker and nondrinker. Family history is positive for OA.

Pt.'s goals: Return to previous level of function and RTW ASAP. Learn to ambulate with crutches

O: Systems review: CV: HR: 84 bpm, BP 124/68, RR 12; edema present in left wrist and ankle; Systems review revealed deficits in the musculoskeletal, neuromuscular, and integumentary systems, see below; Pt. is alert and oriented x 4.

Range of motion: AROM: (R) UE and LE are WNL; (L) shoulder, elbow, and hip are WNL; (L) hand: Pt. can perform a full fist but it is difficult because of edema; (L) Thumb IP, MCP, and CMC joints are WNL.

Knee ROM			
	(L) knee AROM (degrees)	(L) knee PROM (degrees)	(R) knee AROM (degrees)
	0-100	0-110	15-0-145

Wrist ROM			
	(L) wrist AROM (degrees)	(L) wrist PROM (degrees)	(R) wrist AROM (degrees)
Flexion	20	25	90
Extension	10	15	75
UD	10	15	35
RD	10	15	25
Supination	30	35	85
Pronation	40	45	75

Ankle ROM			
	(L) ankle AROM (degrees)	(L) ankle PROM (degrees)	(R) ankle AROM (degrees)
DF	−10 (from neutral)	0	20
PF	20	25	50
Inversion	5	5	50
Eversion	0	5	10

Strength: (R) UE & LE 5/5; (L) shoulder and hip 4/5; (L) elbow, wrist, knee, & ankle deferred because of acuity

Girth: Wrist figure 8 (R): 46 cm (L): 47.2 cm; ankle figure 8 (R): 52 cm (L): 54.1 cm

Sensation: (L) wrist and ankle intact to light touch and (=) when compared to the right

Circulation: 2+ at radial & dorsal pedal arteries on the (L)

Special tests: N/A at this time due to acuity

Gait: Unable to ambulate at this time

Transfers: (I) Bed to/from chair, chair to/from toilet, sit to/from stand all NWB on (L) LE

Bed mobility: (I) All areas.

Today's intervention and home instruction: AAROM for (L) wrist: flexion, extension, pronation, & supination to increase mobility; (L) ankle: DF and PF (also instructed in using opposite foot for self PROM) to increase mobility needed for gait; performed AROM for all digits and thumb to improve grip and decrease edema (15 minutes); instructed pt. in using ice ×20 minutes, elevation, and compression wrapping for ankle and wrist; instructed pt. in use of crutches with platform for (L) UE, PWB 50% on (L) LE using step to gait pattern. Pt. required CGA ×1 for balance with crutches and gait pattern and verbal cueing (30 minutes). Pt. performed all ex. (I) & verbalized understanding of all precautions. Total treatment time 45 minutes following exam.

A: 27 y.o. RHD male 4 wks s/p fall sustaining (L) wrist and ankle fractures. Patient demonstrates impaired mobility and strength in the (L) UE and LE, and edema all limiting his ability to ambulate, drive, work, and manage his family and home tasks.

Problem list: Decreased AROM, PROM, strength, unable to ambulate, unable to perform (I) self-care or home management tasks, and unable to work at this time.

Rehab potential: Pt. demonstrates good potential for full recovery. No comorbidities that could affect outcome identified at this time.

Anticipated goals and expected outcomes:

At the end of 2 weeks, the pt. will:

1. Increase AROM 10 to 15 degrees for the wrist, forearm, and ankle to allow improved mobility and self-care

2. Decrease edema by .5 cm for the wrist and ankle to allow improved mobility

3. Ambulate for unlimited distances with (L) UE platform PWB (L) LE (I)

4. Perform all self-care (I)

5. Perform a full fist without limitations to allow full grip during ADL and self-care

At the end of 12 weeks (d/c), the pt. will:

1. Have normal AROM of the wrist, forearm, & ankle (90-100% of opposite)

2. Grip & pinch strength will be 80-100% of (R)

3. Be (I) with all self-care and home management tasks

4. Ambulate (I) on all surfaces without an assistive device

5. Ascend/descend stairs (I) without an assistive device

6. Drive without restrictions

7. RTW at previous level of employment

P: Skilled services necessary to instruct pt. in safe and appropriate therapeutic exercise, use of assistive device, and gait pattern; also needed to safely progress gait and UE activity as ordered. Also will require instruction in strengthening exercises and retraining in functional mobility to prepare for return to normal lifestyle and RTW. See pt. 2-3×/wk for next 3 months for therapeutic exercise to improve mobility and strength for the hip, knee, shoulder, and elbow; gait training to increase (I) functional mobility to allow return to normal activities and participation. Will progress pt. as tolerated & according to physician orders. Pt. is in agreement with the above stated plan.

John Smith, PT

REFERENCES

1. Quinn L, Gordon J. *Functional Outcomes: Documentation for Rehabilitation.* 2nd ed. Maryland Heights, MO: Saunders Elsevier; 2010.

2. Weed LL. *Medical Records, Medical Education, and Patient Care: The Problem-Oriented Medical Record as a Basic Tool.* Chicago, IL: Year Book Medical Publishers; 1970.

3. Wright A, Sittig DF, McGowan J, Ash JS, Weed LL. Bringing science to medicine: an interview with larry weed, inventor of the problem-oriented medical record. *J Am Med Inform Assoc.* 2014;21:964-968.

4. Dinsdale SM, Mossman PL, Gullickson G, Anderson TP. The problem-oriented medical record in rehabilitation. *Arch Phys Med Rehabil.* 1970;51:488-492.

5. Milhous RL. The problem-oriented medical record in rehabilitation management and training. *Arch Phys Med Rehabil.* 1972;53:182-185.

6. Feinstein AR. The problems of the "problem-oriented medical record." *Ann Intern Med.* 1973;78:751-762.

7. Mcintyre N. The problem-oriented medical record. *Br Med J.* 1973;2:598-600.

8. Reinstein L. Problem-oriented medical record: experience in 238 rehabilitation institutions. *Arch Phys Med Rehabil.* 1977;58:398-401.

9. Echternach JL. Use of the problem oriented clinical note in a physical therapy department. *Phys Ther.* 1974;54:19-22.

10. Reinstein L, Staas WE, Marquette CH. A rehabilitation evaluation system which complements the problem-oriented medical record. *Arch Phys Med Rehabil.* 1975;56:396-399.

11. Abeln SH. Improving functional reporting. *PT Magazine.* 1996;4(3):26, 28-30.

12. Centers for Medicare and Medicaid Services. Minimum Data Set 3.0 public records. https://www.cms.gov/Research-Statistics-Data-and-Systems/Computer-Data-and-Systems/Minimum-Data-Set-3-0-Public-Reports/index.html. Accessed April 3, 2019.

13. Centers for Medicare and Medicaid Services. Inpatient rehabilitation facility PPS. https://www.cms.gov/Medicare/Medicare-Fee-for-Service-Payment/InpatientRehabFacPPS/index.html?redirect=/InpatientRehabFacPPS/01_overview.asp updated 4/16/2013. Published 2013. Accessed April 3, 2019.

14. Centers for Medicare and Medicaid Services. Home health PPS. https://www.cms.gov/Medicare/Medicare-Fee-for-Service-Payment/HomeHealthPPS/index.html. Published May. Accessed April 3, 2019.

15. Individuals with Disabilities in Education Act of 2004, PL 108-446. 108th Congress (2004). https://ies.ed.gov/ncser/pdf/pl108-446.pdf Accessed April 3, 2019.

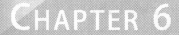

CHAPTER 6

Health Informatics and Electronic Health Records

Ralph R. Utzman, PT, MPH, PhD

CHAPTER OUTLINE

- Health Informatics, Health Information Technology, and Physical Therapy Practice
- The Evolution of Electronic Health Records
- Electronic Health Records in Physical Therapy Practice
  - Benefits of Electronic Documentation for Physical Therapists
  - Challenges in Electronic Health Records
  - Tips for Documenting in Electronic Health Records
- Electronic Documentation and Clinical Outcomes

CHAPTER OBJECTIVES

Upon completion of this chapter, the reader will be able to:

1. Define health informatics, health information, health information technology, interoperability, and clinical outcomes registry
2. Describe ways in which physical therapists use health information technology in clinical practice
3. Differentiate between electronic medical records and electronic health records
4. List the 5 priorities of the Department of Health and Human Services in developing "meaningful use" requirements for the adoption of electronic health records
5. Discuss considerations for adopting and using electronic health records in physical therapy practice
6. Give examples of prompts and decision support provided by EHR systems
7. Discuss potential benefits and challenges presented by EHRs
8. List tips for documenting in electronic medical records
9. Discuss ways in which physical therapists should be involved in developing and refining EHR systems

Erickson ML, Utzman RR, McKnight RS.
*Physical Therapy Documentation: From Examination to Outcome,
Third Edition* (pp 53-60).
© 2020 Taylor & Francis Group.

KEY TERMS

clinical outcomes registry
decision support
electronic health record
electronic medical record
health informatics
health information
health information technology
interoperability

KEY ABBREVIATIONS

EHR
EMR
HIT
HITECH Act

Advances in technology and practice over the past 2 decades have transformed how physical therapists document patient care. Traditionally, physical therapists documented care via chronological, handwritten notations on paper that were filed in folders or binders. In hospitals and other large facilities, these "charts" included notes from multiple health care providers and workers. Because of the physical nature of the medical record, it was impossible for multiple providers, even those working in the same facility, to work with a patient's "chart" at the same time. The paper medical record was a passive repository of information that was often illegible and/or recorded in an unstandardized fashion. Extracting data for quality improvement or research purposes was difficult and expensive. Sharing information with patients, payers, and other stakeholders required photocopying and mailing reams of paper.

Today's electronic health records (EHRs) are designed to overcome the shortcomings of paper-based records. In many facilities, a patient's record can be viewed and edited by multiple personnel at once. Electronic documentation systems can help structure and focus data entry while providing reminders and prompts to clinicians. Coding and storage of information are increasingly standardized, making searching, retrieval, and transmission faster and easier. Patient care data are now stored on electronic media and/or "in the cloud" instead of bulky physical files.

Like other health care providers, physical therapists must manage large amounts of information in order to care for patients. This chapter introduces the reader to EHRs, as well as the larger context of health informatics.

HEALTH INFORMATICS, HEALTH INFORMATION TECHNOLOGY, AND PHYSICAL THERAPIST PRACTICE

Health informatics refers to the science of collecting, storing, retrieving, and using medical, health, and patient information. The term also refers to an emerging, interdisciplinary field of study in health care, bringing together expertise in health information technology (HIT), engineering, business, finance, and health care. A broad goal of health informatics is to improve integration and communication within the health care system to improve safety and outcomes.[1] Health information refers to all the data related to a person's health and medical history, including symptoms, diagnoses, treatments, and outcomes. HIT refers to the application of technology to manage health and patient information.

Today's physical therapist interacts with HIT every day. The following are some examples:

- A physical therapist seeking scientific evidence on the most appropriate treatment for a patient with an unfamiliar diagnosis searches online databases, such as PubMed, for citations of peer-reviewed articles. Once relevant articles are identified, the physical therapist accesses digital copies of those articles for review. The physical therapist also consults other online sources for evidence-based practice, such as the Cochrane Database of Systematic Reviews or the Physiotherapy Evidence Database.

- Before coming to the clinic, a patient is asked to complete an online intake questionnaire.

- The physical therapist uses a computer terminal or tablet computer to access the patient's medical history, referral, and intake questionnaire before seeing the patient.

- During the care of the patient, the physical therapist enters the history and examination data into a computer terminal or tablet computer.

- The physical therapist performs computerized testing of the patient's balance using dynamic posturography. Measurements of the patient's balance are transmitted to and stored in the patient's medical record.

- Following the patient encounter, the physical therapist completes documentation regarding the patient's visit and enters charges for the visit. These charges are converted electronically to *Current Procedural Terminology* codes. These codes are used to generate a bill that is electronically transmitted to the patient's insurance company. (See Chapter 12 for more about coding and billing.)

- A physical therapist is creating a therapeutic exercise program for a patient to carry out at home. The physical therapist uses a web-based program to generate instructions for each exercise the patient is to perform. The physical therapist prints a hard copy of the instructions to review with the patient. The software also generates an electronic copy of the instructions that is emailed to the patient. The emailed instructions include links to online video demonstrations the patient can access from his or her home computer.

- A physical therapist is working with a group of colleagues on a quality improvement project. He or she wants to find out why the clinic has experienced an increase in patient "no shows" over the past 6 months. Working with the facility's HIT staff, he or she pulls aggregate data from the EHR regarding the patient diagnosis, referral source, therapist, visit frequency, and other relevant details for analysis.
- A physical therapist receives quarterly reports from a clinical outcomes registry. The report compares the outcomes of the physical therapist's patients with those of therapists at other similar facilities.

Clearly, the physical therapist is not expected to be an expert in HIT. However, in order to effectively care for patients in the 21st century, physical therapists have to be fluent in using technology to manage patient health information. To accomplish this, physical therapists need to routinely consult and collaborate with experts in various health informatics fields.

THE EVOLUTION OF ELECTRONIC HEALTH RECORDS

Electronic medical record (EMR) and EHR are often used interchangeably; however, the terms represent different concepts. The EMR is defined as an electronic record of the patient's health information that exists within a single practice, hospital, or health system.[2] Patients may have access to view portions of the EMR through an online portal but cannot interact with their data record. In contrast, the EHR is an electronic record that is shared across organizations.[2] In order for an EHR to incorporate data from multiple care delivery organizations, EHR systems must be interoperable (ie, hardware and software must be designed according to specific standards so that different EHR systems can "talk to each other" and share data).[2]

In 2004, President George W. Bush launched a broad initiative to expand HIT in the United States. He created the Office of the National Coordinator for HIT, and Dr. David Brailer was named the first Office of the National Coordinator for HIT chief. President Bush's goal was to give all Americans access to their own personal EHR within 10 years.[3] Despite this ambitious goal, the initiative received little funding.[3] In 2009, President Barack Obama signed the American Recovery and Reinvestment Act. This legislation included the Health Information Technology

for Economic and Clinical Health (HITECH) Act, which provided financial incentives to eligible health care providers who demonstrate "meaningful use" of certified EHR systems.[3] The HITECH Act provided significantly more funding and accompanying regulations to support the expansion of EHRs. At least $35 billion in taxpayer funds have been allocated to the initiative.[4,5]

As of this writing, the HITECH Act financial incentives are only available to hospitals, critical access hospitals, and physicians.[6] Physical therapists in private practices, home health agencies, and skilled nursing facilities are not eligible for the financial incentives to support the adoption and development of EHRs. However, because physical therapists in these settings communicate and interact with hospitals and physicians who are eligible, physical therapists have had to adopt electronic documentation systems that are interoperable and meet "meaningful use" standards.[6]

The "meaningful use" rules were developed by the US Department of Health and Human Services and focus on 5 health policy priorities[7]:

1. Improve quality, safety, and efficiency and reduce health disparities
2. Engage patients and families in their health
3. Improve coordination of care
4. Improve population and public health
5. Ensure privacy and security of health information

The regulations were implemented in 3 stages. Going forward, compliance with the "meaningful use" regulations has been incorporated into the Medicare Incentive Payment Program for eligible providers. Hospitals and physicians who are in compliance will continue to receive incentive payments; those who are not in compliance will face payment reductions and other financial penalties. The American Physical Therapy Association continues to advocate for the inclusion of physical therapists in private practice and other excluded settings to be incorporated into the meaningful use program.[8]

ELECTRONIC HEALTH RECORDS IN PHYSICAL THERAPY PRACTICE

Health care organizations, including physical therapy practices, have many options when choosing an EHR system. In a traditional server-client model, the organization purchases a central computer, or server, to house the EHR software.[9] The organization also purchases terminal computers that are linked to the main server. The clinician uses these terminals to access the software and patient records. This type of system is expensive due to the costs of the hardware, software, and technical support needed to set up and maintain it. On the other end of the spectrum, some practices choose to adopt a web-based EHR program.[9] In these types of systems, the organization subscribes to

Figure 6-1. Sample electronic documentation.

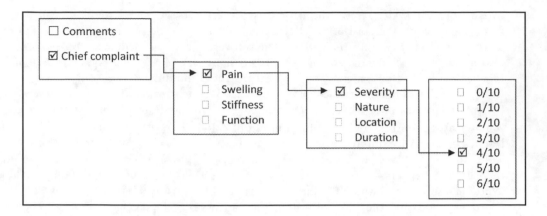

Figure 6-2. The hypothetical creations of an electronic note.

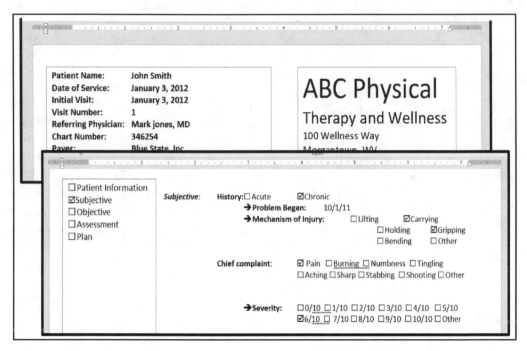

software that runs in a web browser. The organization can use PCs, laptops, and, in some cases, tablet computers to access the software. Web-based EHR systems require less equipment and are thus less expensive to set up and maintain. However, the patient's data are housed externally by a third party instead of on a central computer owned and housed by the organization.[9]

In addition to where the EHR hardware and software are housed, the organization must decide how different software systems will integrate with each other. Organizations may purchase a packaged "suite" that brings together patient admission/registration, scheduling, ordering, documentation, and billing functions in one package. Another approach is to purchase separate software to handle each of these functions. This approach allows the organization to pick the best systems, perhaps from different vendors, to handle specific practice needs. The challenge of the "best-of-breed" approach is that the various systems have to be able to share information with each other. For example, data collected into the patient registration software will need to be passed on to the software used for scheduling

and documentation, and those systems need to share information with the software used for billing.

Physical therapists may use a variety of documentation systems and methods across health settings. Physical therapists may complete their documentation using computer terminals in fixed locations, laptops or other portable computers on mobile carts, or tablets or other small handheld devices. Data are typically entered using a traditional mouse and keyboard or via touch screen. Some systems allow clinicians to dictate their notes, and transcription software converts the recorded speech into printed text. If information is captured on paper, the document can be scanned, converted into a digital format, and uploaded to the patient's record. Many EHR systems allow digital images to be imported, and some will store video files.

Electronic documentation software packages in physical therapy typically present the clinician with electronic forms or templates based on body systems or regions. These templates incorporate checkboxes, pull-down menus, and other time-saving features (Figures 6-1 and 6-2). Rather than enter information in a free-form, narrative note, documentation is organized according to the template form. Software packages contain ways to document a variety of note types including initial documentation, interim notes, progress notes, and discharge summaries. Like paper forms, electronic templates are used to standardize terminology, structure, and contents of documentation between patients and clinicians and to improve communication throughout an organization. Standards for EHR software (such as HL7, Health Level Seven International) continue to evolve to ensure data are stored in a way that contributes to interoperability. However, within this standardization, a level of flexibility for the needs of various health care providers can and should be achieved because all patient cases may not fit into the standard template. Documentation software should have flexibility for the development of templates that will match the needs of different settings and patients. Some software packages can generate special types of documentation such as letters, progress reports, and flow sheets populated with previously recorded data with a few clicks, and this can be a significant time-saving benefit for clinicians. Other benefits are the ability to track the number of visits and insurance authorization. It also allows the clinicians or office staff to set prompts designed to remind the physical therapist and physical therapist assistant when various processes need to occur such as reassessments, plan of care updates, and insurance recertification.

Prompts and decision support provided by the EHR can assist physical therapists in efficiently producing complete and accurate records of patient care. Prompts embedded within electronic forms may remind the clinician to collect and record important information. For example, when a physical therapist creates documentation of an initial patient visit, the software may prompt him or her to include the patient's medical diagnosis and the date of onset. The system may force the physical therapist to enter certain data before continuing or completing the note. Some form fields may be formatted to require the entry of specific types of data. For example, an electronic flow sheet for entering vital signs may force the clinician to enter numeric data rather than text. As computer hardware and software become more powerful, EHR systems are able to provide increasingly more sophisticated decision support. For example, if a physical therapist enters a notation indicating the patient reports symptoms of dizziness, the EHR may prompt the therapist to consider performing an examination of the patient's oculomotor function and balance.

EHRs are big business. Numerous companies, large and small, provide EHR software and hardware that are used in different settings. It is beyond the scope of this textbook to provide an exhaustive review of the myriad of systems available. Throughout a Doctor of Physical Therapy student's clinical education, the student may use a different documentation system for each clinical experience. The author recommends students become fluent in the basic principles and practices of documentation; those skills can be adapted for use in various EHR systems.

Benefits of Electronic Documentation for Physical Therapists

As noted previously, EHR systems hold many advantages compared with traditional paper-based documentation methods. Electronic documentation produces more legible, complete, and accurate records.[2,10,11] In an EHR, the patient's record is more accessible to the physical therapists, other clinicians, and the patient.[10,11] Because data can be transferred and shared electronically rather than via photocopying, faxing, and mailing, EHRs enhance communication between the physical therapist and other members of the health care team.[10,11] In paper-based systems, physical therapists often have to rewrite data as they compile patient progress reports for referring physicians, insurers, and others. The EHR allows the physical therapist to enter information once and then use that data later in reports and other documents.[2,10] Having test results and other information entered into the EHR by the health care team, along with clinical decision support systems, enhances clinicians' abilities to make timely clinical decisions.[2] Because of these many benefits, EHRs have the potential to increase clinician efficiency and productivity while reducing waste of time and other resources.[2,10,11] This can ultimately lead to cost savings and improve health outcomes.[2,11]

Challenges in Electronic Health Records

The use of EHRs in the United States has grown dramatically in the past decade. In a pilot survey of nearly 7000 physical therapists conducted in 2016, two thirds reported using an EHR system for at least part of their practice.[2] Between 2004 and 2017, the use of EHRs by physicians rose from 21% to 86%.[12] From 2008 to 2017, the use of EHRs by hospitals rose from 10% to 96%.[13] Despite the numerous potential benefits of EHRs, the rapid transition to electronic systems has presented some challenges and pitfalls.

A recent article published in *Fortune*[5] magazine outlines several concerning trends. First, the authors identify cases in which EHR systems caused or contributed to errors in patient care, some of which were fatal. Second, they cite cases in which providers have taken advantage of EHR software to commit insurance fraud and abuse. Third, they highlight problems with system interoperability (eg, one software/hardware system not correctly interfacing with another).[5]

Despite the goal of providing patients with access to their own medical information, Fry and Schulte[5] suggest the security and confidentiality features used by EHR systems instead create significant barriers to patients gaining access. Back in the days of paper records, the security and confidentiality of a patient's health information were maintained primarily by limiting physical access to the patient's chart. The goal of making data more accessible through the adoption of EHRs has made security and confidentiality much more complicated. Organizations that deliver health care are required by federal Health Insurance Portability and Accountability Act and HITECH regulations to enforce strict policies for security and confidentiality and to monitor for and respond to breaches.[14] Today's sophisticated EHR systems are able to create audit trails to show exactly who accessed each patient's record, what information they accessed, and when they accessed it.[14] However, passwords can be stolen, digital systems can be hacked, and humans who use these complex information systems make mistakes due to carelessness, poor training, fatigue, and poor system design.[5,14] Striking a balance between making information accessible and making information secure continues to be a significant EHR challenge.

One of the potential benefits of EHR adoptions is increased time efficiency and reduced administrative burden for clinicians.[11] However, Fry and Schulte[5] provide statistics that suggest the adoption of EHR has increased the workload of many health care providers. Recent studies of physicians suggest this increased administrative workload may contribute to practitioner burnout. According to a recent survey, the average primary care physicians spend 6 hours per day working in EHR systems.[15] Another study of physicians found that for every hour of direct patient care, physicians spend up to 2 hours working in the EMR.[16] Many physicians report spending an hour or 2 at home each evening to complete their administrative work.[5,16] A recent national report on physician depression and burnout found alarming rates of physician burnout (28% to 54% depending on specialty).[17] Nearly 60% of survey respondents cited administrative tasks, such as documentation, as the factor that most contributes to burnout.[17]

What does this mean for physical therapists and student physical therapists? First, we must develop good documentation skills that do not rely solely on technology. Being able to organize data collected and generated during patient care and to articulate the rationale for clinical decisions in writing are fundamental skills for all health care providers. Regardless of the EHR system used, inaccurate or incomplete documentation can lead to patient safety issues and/or accusations of fraud and abuse (see Chapter 3). Second, we must be willing and able to collaborate with those who develop, design, and deploy EHRs and other HIT systems we use in clinical practice. Physical therapist practice is unique in many ways from the practice of physicians, nurses, and other health professionals. Our voices are vital in making sure EHR systems used in physical therapy are useful, safe, and efficient. Third, physical therapists need to engage in research to clarify how EHRs are impacting our own workflow and practice patterns, how to optimize the benefits of EHRs, and how to overcome challenges presented by EHRs. Finally, we must participate in advocacy efforts by the American Physical Therapy Association to address administrative burdens that detract from care provided by physical therapists.

Tips for Documenting in Electronic Health Records

1. Avoid cloned notes. EHR software makes it possible to copy and paste information from one document to another. Some clinicians overuse this capability, "cloning" daily notes so that each note looks the same. The American Health Information Management Association recommends health care organizations (including those where physical therapists practice) develop clear policies and procedures regarding the acceptable use of "cut and paste" features within the EHR.[18] When the same content is repeated within daily notes across multiple patient visits, the documentation does not accurately demonstrate skilled services were provided, which may lead insurers to deny payment for services.[19]

2. Avoid repetitive charting habits. Besides cloning notes, the overuse of flow sheets and drop-down lists can also make documentation look repetitive. Be sure to use open text fields to concisely "tell the story" of the patient's care.[19]

3. Develop templates and forms that match your patient caseload. Using documentation templates that do not match your patient can be time consuming because you need to make modifications and add more text to accurately describe the patient's condition, movement, and the care provided. Although it is not reasonable to have a perfect form or template to fit every patient encounter, developing templates for common patient diagnoses and visit types can help you save time while making your documentation more accurate and complete.

4. Use software features to produce reports and letters. Physical therapists often generate letters to update referring physicians and other team members on their patients' care and progress. In addition, third-party payers often require care plans and progress reports to authorize insurance payment for services provided. Many EHR systems have features to create letters and reports that pull data from examination or daily treatment notes. Using these features can help save time by eliminating the need to extract information that was already entered into the record and rewriting the reports.

5. Develop and enable helpful software prompts and cues. As noted earlier, EHR software's decision support capabilities are gradually becoming more sophisticated. The judicious use of these features can help improve care quality and safety and encourage more complete documentation. However, too many prompts can lead to "alert fatigue,"[5] so work with your practice

administration and HIT staff/vendors to optimize these features to fit your practice/organization.

6. Focus on function, medical necessity, and skilled care. Regardless of the documentation technology and methods used, defensible documentation demonstrates why the patient needs physical therapy and why those services require the skills of a physical therapist.[20] Make sure you are using the best outcome measures to document the patient's function (see Chapter 11), and paint a picture of how the patient's function is affected by their health condition. Then, describe how the services provided address the patient's function and why those services require the knowledge and expertise of a physical therapist. In the EHR, clinicians will often need to use a combination of form fields and free-text boxes to capture this information.

7. Be part of the solution. As noted earlier, EHR technology still has a long way to go. Engage in quality improvement projects and other initiatives to find ways to better leverage technology to support physical therapist practice.

ELECTRONIC DOCUMENTATION AND CLINICAL OUTCOMES

Chapter 11 presents the concepts of measuring and documenting patient outcomes. The end of the chapter outlines steps for developing a plan for assessing outcomes in your practice. Chapter 12 discusses reimbursement for the care of our services, including the transition toward value-based payment models that focus on outcomes and efficiency. EHRs can provide tools for collecting, tracking, analyzing, and reporting clinical outcomes. These tools can assist in demonstrating the effectiveness and efficiency of your services and in justifying appropriate payment for those services.

Clinical outcomes registries are an emerging EHR tool being adopted in physical therapist practices in the United States. To use an outcomes registry, the physical therapy practice or organization subscribes to be a registry member or participant. The practice or organization then submits information regarding the patient and the patient's care to the registry, such as diagnoses, comorbidities, treatments provided, and measurements on standard outcomes measures.

Clinical data registries can be designated as "qualified" by the Centers for Medicare and Medicaid Services.[21] By reporting patient data to a qualified registry, a practice or organization can meet regulatory requirements for Medicare and Medicaid such as the Medicare Incentive Payment Program (see Chapter 12). Clinical data registries can also report data to other insurance providers as well. Examples of clinical data registries in physical therapy are the American Physical Therapy Association's Physical Therapy Outcomes Registry (http://www.ptoutcomes.com) and FOTO (Focus on Therapeutic Outcomes, https://www.fotoinc.com/). Besides providing information to insurance companies for payment, the use of an outcomes registry provides a physical therapy clinic or practice with benchmarking information (ie, the clinic or practice can compare their outcomes and efficiency with other similar clinics/practices). This information can be used to educate clinicians, improve documentation, drive quality improvement within the practice, and market the practice to patients, referral sources, and insurers.[22,23]

SUMMARY

Documentation is an essential skill for all physical therapists. Doing it well, regardless of the system or technology, can enhance patient care, promote optional patient outcomes, and support appropriate payment for services provided by physical therapists. As the use of EHRs continues to progress, physical therapists must take an active role in developing, selecting, implementing, and improving the systems used in their practices. We must engage in health services research and quality improvement projects to establish, promote, and adopt best practices for the documentation of care. We must collaborate with experts in health informatics and HIT to develop systems of the future that will deliver on the promise of secure EHRs that support our clinical practices, facilitate team communication, and empower patients to participate in their health care.

REFERENCES

1. American Medical Informatics Association. What is informatics? American Medical Informatics Association website. https://www.amia.org/fact-sheets/what-informatics. Accessed May 1, 2019.

2. American Physical Therapy Association. Understanding and adopting electronic health records: part 1 - decision. APTA website. http://www.apta.org/EHR/Guide/Decision/. Updated May 8, 2016. Accessed May 1, 2019.

3. Conn J. 10 years afer the revolution: health IT coordinators look back a the nation's progress. Modern Healthcare website. https://www.modernhealthcare.com/article/20140405/MAGAZINE/304059980/10-years-after-the-revolution. Updated April 5, 2014. Accessed May 2, 2019.

4. Thune J, Alexander L, Roberts P, Burr R, Enzi M. Where is HITECH's $35 billion dollar investment going? *Health Affairs Blog.* March 4, 2015. https://www.healthaffairs.org/do/10.1377/hblog20150304.045199/full/. Accessed May 1, 2019.

5. Fry E, Schulte F. Death by a thousand clicks. *Fortune.* 2019;179(4):56-73.

6. American Physical Therapy Association. Electronic health records (EHR). APTA website. https://www.apta.org/EHR/. Updated May 18, 2016. Accessed May 1, 2019.

7. Centers for Disease Control and Prevention. Meaningful use. Public Health and Promoting Interoperability Programs website. https://www.cdc.gov/ehrmeaningfuluse/introduction.html. Updated January 18, 2017. Accessed May 1, 2019.

8. Dunn SL. Letter to Don Rucker, National Coordinator for Health Information Technology. APTA website. http://www.apta.org/uploadedFiles/APTAorg/Advocacy/Federal/Legislative_Issues/Health_IT/Comments/APTAComments_StrategyReducingRegulatoryAdministrativeBurdenHealthITEHRs.pdf. Updated January 22, 2019. Accessed May 1, 2019.

9. American Physical Therapy Association. Understanding and adopting electronic health records: part 3 - selection. APTA website. http://www.apta.org/EHR/Guide/Selection/. Updated May 18, 2016. Accessed May 1, 2019.

10. Vreeman DJ, Taggard SL, Rhine MD, Worrell TW. Evidence for electronic health record systems in physical therapy. *Phys Ther.* 2006;86(3):434-446; discussion 446-439.

11. Office of the National Coordinator for Health Information Technology. What are the advantages of electronic health records? US Department of Health & Human Services. https://www.healthit.gov/faq/what-are-advantages-electronic-health-records. Updated November 9, 2018. Accessed May 1, 2019.

12. Office of the National Coordinator for Health Information Technology. Ofice-based physician electronic health record adoption. Health IT Quick-Stat #50 website. https://dashboard.healthit.gov/quickstats/pages/physician-ehr-adoption-trends.php. Updated January 2019. Accessed.

13. Office of the National Coordinator for Health Information Technology. Non-federal acute care hospital electronic health record adoption. Health IT Quick-Stat #47 website. https://dashboard.healthit.gov/quickstats/pages/FIG-Hospital-EHR-Adoption.php. Updated September 2017. Accessed.

14. Harman LB, Flite CA, Bond K. Electronic health records: privacy, confidentiality, and security. *Virtual Mentor.* 2012;14(9):712-719.

15. Arndt BG, Beasley JW, Watkinson MD, et al. Tethered to the EHR: primary care physician workload assessment using EHR event log data and time-motion observations. *Ann Fam Med.* 2017;15(5):419-426.

16. Sinsky C, Colligan L, Li L, et al. Allocation of physician time in ambulatory practice: a time and motion study in 4 specialties. *Ann Intern Med.* 2016;165(11):753-760.

17. Kane L. Medscape national physician burnout, depression & suicide report 2019. Medscape website. https://www.medscape.com/2019-lifestyle-burnout. Updated January 16, 2019. Accessed May 1, 2019.

18. American Health Information Management Association. Appropriate use of the copy and paste functionality in electronic health records. AHIMA website. http://bok.ahima.org/PdfView?oid=300306. Updated March 17, 2014. Accessed May 1, 2019.

19. Evans WK. Keys to effective documentation: be thorough and think like a payer. *PT in Motion.* 2016;8(7):8-12.

20. Diedrich D, Warhsauer J. Tell your patient's story: tips for defensible documentation. APTA #PTTransforms Blog website. http://www.apta.org/Blogs/PTTransforms/2019/5/7/TellYourPatientsStory/. Updated May 7, 2019. Accessed May 7, 2019.

21. Centers for Medicare & Mediciaid Services. Brief overview of qualified clinical data registries. Measure Management & You website. https://www.cms.gov/Medicare/Quality-Initiatives-Patient-Assessment-Instruments/MMS/Downloads/A-Brief-Overview-of-Qualified-Clinical-Data-Registries.pdf. Updated October 2018. Accessed May 1, 2019.

22. Vanderhoff M. Strength in numbers: the power and potential of clinical data registries. *PT in Motion.* 2017;9(10):34-38.

23. American Physical Therapy Association. Physical therapy outcomes registry. PT Outcomes Registry website. http://www.ptoutcomes.com/home.aspx. Accessed May 1, 2019.

CHAPTER 7

Rules for Writing in Medical Records

Mia L. Erickson, PT, EdD

CHAPTER OUTLINE

- Rules for Writing

CHAPTER OBJECTIVES

Upon completion of this chapter, the reader will be able to:
1. Apply basic rules for documenting in medical records
2. Describe what is meant by "unsubstantiated" terms written in a note
3. Describe the importance of using skilled, medical language in medical records
4. List ways to make notes more readable by others
5. Correctly document late entries and addendums
6. Correct errors written in a medical record

Erickson ML, Utzman RR, McKnight RS.
Physical Therapy Documentation: From Examination to Outcome,
Third Edition (pp 61-67).
© 2020 Taylor & Francis Group.

KEY TERMS

addendum
authenticate
late entry

KEY ABBREVIATIONS

EMR

RULES FOR WRITING

Keep medical records secure. Keep paper medical records and patient information in a secure, fireproof, locked file. Password protect and securely store electronic records to prevent unauthorized access. Use laptops, tablets, or computers in a manner in which they are not viewable by others or use privacy screen filters. Set computers to "time-out" after a period of nonuse.

Authenticate all entries. Date and authenticate (sign) all notations made in a patient's medical record, paper or electronic. In most cases, any individual who participates in the care of the patient/client should sign the documentation. State regulations often dictate whose signature should appear in the record. Often, the provider's credentials and license number should also be included. This is also dictated by state regulations. The physical therapist authenticates the initial examination, evaluation, diagnosis, prognosis, and intervention plan. The physical therapist and/or the physical therapist assistant (where permissible by law) authenticate the treatment notes, and the physical therapist authenticates the progress reports and discharge summaries. Electronic signatures are also acceptable.

All records should be complete. Place all relevant information related to the patient/client in his or her medical record. Include the patient's name, parent or guardian information (for minors), address, date of birth, health insurance information, emergency contact information, and physician information. Include all documentation reflecting the episode of care, such as consent forms, intake forms (eg, prior medical history and self-report questionnaires), initial documentation, interim notes, progress reports following regular reassessments, re-evaluations when performed, discharge summaries, physician referrals, letters, communication notes, referrals to other health care providers, flow sheets, home exercise programs, and any other pertinent information related to the episode of care. Include attachments such as digital images or video. In a hospital setting,

---

Example 7-1. Outpatient Cancellation Note

In an outpatient clinic, a snowstorm in December caused a patient to miss 2 appointments. Document:

12/19/19: Mrs. Smith canceled her appointment because of weather. Rescheduled for 12/21.

Sue Brooks, PT

12/21/19: Mrs. Smith canceled her appointment because of weather. Rescheduled for 12/23.

Sue Brooks, PT

Example 7-2. Inpatient Cancellation Note

On a skilled nursing unit, the nurse asks that you not work with a patient because the physician suspects the patient has a blood clot and is awaiting a Doppler study. Document:

12/12/19: Attempted to see Mrs. Smith this morning; however, nursing asked that we hold therapy because of possible blood clot, awaiting Doppler study. Will resume when cleared.

Sue Brooks, PT

---

where all providers document in one medical record, one will find documentation completed by physicians, nurses, and other providers, as well as things such as lab reports and imaging studies. Document special circumstances or situations in the patient's medical record such as cancellations and missed appointments. Document reasons for canceled or missed appointments or treatment sessions whether initiated by the patient, the physical therapist or physical therapist assistant, or another health care provider (Examples 7-1 and 7-2).

Document all telephone or electronic conversations, such as email, related to patient care (Examples 7-3 and 7-4). This could include conversations with the patent, the patient's family/caregiver, the physician, other health care providers, or case managers.

There may be times when the physician (or physician assistant) provides an order over the phone or in person. Document verbal orders as shown in Example 7-5.

The physician giving the verbal order then signs the order as soon as possible. It is important to note that

Example 7-3. Telephone Call 1

You are working with a 24-year-old who was injured in a workplace accident. The patient's case manager for worker's compensation contacts you to determine the patient's status and progress. Document:

12/22/19: Spoke with pt.'s case manager today and provided update on strength, ROM, and functional status as of reassessment performed on 12/20/19.

Sue Brooks, PT

Example 7-4. Telephone Call 2

You are working with a patient with Alzheimer disease who has recently undergone a right tibial open reduction and internal fixation because of a fracture. The orthopedic physician ordered "gait training non-weight bearing (R) LE." However, because of the patient's confusion and inability to follow commands, she is unable to maintain these weight-bearing restrictions. You call the physician to make him aware of the situation. Document:

12/01/19: Called Dr. Jones to make him aware that Mrs. Smith is unable to maintain weight-bearing restrictions because of confusion and inability to follow commands. Left message with nurse. Hold gait training until speaking with physician.

Sue Brooks, PT

Example 7-5. Verbal Order

1/14/19: Verbal order received from Dr. Haines 1/14/19 @ 1:30 PM: Initiate compression wrap to pt.'s (L) foot.

Sue Brooks, PT

Example 7-6. Unexpected Situation

You are working with a 22-year-old woman who underwent a ligament repair to her right knee. She is performing resisted knee flexion strengthening and felt a "pop" in her knee. She immediately reported an increase in pain from 0/10 to 5/10. Document:

12/12/19: Pt. was performing right knee flexion exercises per standard protocol and felt a "pop" in her knee. Pain increased from 0/10 to 5/10. The pt. was asked to discontinue her exercises for the day. Pt. received ice to the knee for 20 minutes. Called physician and left message with nurse for him to call back. After ice, pt. reported a decrease in pain to 0/10, and she was able to ambulate without a limp. Will speak with physician about whether he wants to see the pt. or continue with therapy.

Sue Brooks, PT

physical therapist assistants do not take verbal orders or interpret referrals to physical therapy. In today's electronic age, verbal orders are rarely taken by physical therapists. Instead, following the communication, the physician writes a new order in the electronic medical record (EMR) or, in an outpatient setting, generates a new prescription or order, and it is transmitted to the therapy office. Document unusual or unexpected situations or outcomes. Some of these situations may also require the creation of an incident report. Risk managers can help in determining if an incident report is needed; this is discussed further in Chapter 3. When an unusual event occurs, document the event, the patient's response in objective and measurable terms, your actions or response, and the outcome (Example 7-6).

Complete documentation tasks in a timely manner. Documentation should be completed as soon as possible after the session. First, the treatment session is fresh in your head, and you are more likely to remember details sooner

rather than later. In addition, timely, completed documentation is necessary so that another therapist can treat your patient in the event of your absence or another health care provider can obtain necessary information related to the patient. There are also administrative reasons for timely documentation. These include filing reimbursement claims and sending progress updates to others involved in the patient's care, including physicians, case managers, or insurance companies. Clinics and hospitals are likely to have policies in place requiring the completion of all patient documentation within a given time frame.

Documentation should be relevant, accurate, and logical. Ensure that entries in the medical record are relevant to the current condition and episode of care, reflect all necessary components of the session, and are presented in a logical manner. Be as accurate as possible when documenting patient/client data and provide the reader with an accurate description of the patient, justification for the skilled care provided, changes in patient status, and upcoming plans. Any clinician should be able to open the patient records,

Example 7-7. Skilled Language 1

DO NOT WRITE:
Pt. performed therapeutic exercise for 15 minutes.
Instead, describe why the patient performed the exercises.
Pt. performed strengthening exercises for the left quadriceps and hamstrings for 15 minutes to improve knee control during gait. Tactile cues were required for quadriceps facilitation.

Example 7-8. Skilled Language 2

DO NOT WRITE:
Pt. ambulated 15 minutes requiring moderate assist of 1.
Instead, document the assist provided during ambulation.
Pt. ambulated 15 minutes requiring moderate assist of 1 to facilitate (R) quadriceps during the swing phase of gait to increase knee extension and step length.

have a clear idea of what happened, and be able to continue with the intervention in your absence.

Document using objective language including facts and observations. Avoid making remarks about patients that cannot be substantiated by objective data. Remarks about a patient's response to a treatment should be given in objective, measurable terms (eg, "Patient's active range of motion increased from 80 to 110 degrees following treatment, allowing the patient to sit more comfortably in a chair."). Avoid comments or assessments about the patient's personality or his or her psychological status, especially when they are outside the physical therapist's scope of practice (eg, "Patient depressed."). Finally, use professional, neutral language, and do not write unnecessary remarks about the patient, family member, caregiver, or another provider. You should not look as though you are taking sides on any issues between the patient and another individual (eg, a physician or case manager). Use proper spelling, language, and grammar. In the EMR, use the spell-check function.

Be clear and concise. Entries must be clear and concise but also be thorough and provide sufficient information to accurately reflect the encounter, demonstrate that services were skilled, and prove that the intervention is reasonable and necessary. Never leave out pertinent information or a rationale for services for the sake of brevity. As you are learning to write medical records, err on the side of being too lengthy or verbose. You can learn to "skim down" later

after you get more experience and better understand the required information.

Be consistent with your documentation format. This rule largely applies to those using paper-based medical records because the EMR provides consistent templates and forms. In general, use similar types of documentation throughout the patient's episode of care (eg, forms, templates, formats, and flow sheets). Use a similar format or template for documenting all body parts or diagnoses. Also, use similar formats or templates for writing interim notes, progress reports, re-evaluations, and discharge summaries so that reviewers and other health care providers can easily locate necessary information. It also helps another physical therapist or physical therapist assistant find information quickly.

Handwritten entries should be legible. Handwriting that is not legible has the potential to lead to medical errors. In addition, third-party payers have been known to deny claims based solely on the fact that they could not read the provider's handwriting. If this is a problem, consider dictating your notes and using a transcription service or converting to an EMR.

Document using scientific, clinically appropriate language. In most cases, use professional, scientific, medical terminology. Avoid "nonskilled language" such as "the patient walked …." Instead, use descriptive, functional, or medical language, such as "provided gait and transfer training …" or "the patient ambulated …." However, there may be times when more lay language is appropriate. This might be during a pediatric, school-based session where a copy of the documentation is provided to the parents or guardians at the end of the day.

Document the unique skills provided to the patient. Describe the unique skills or assist used or provided to facilitate the patient during the session(s) that go above and beyond what could be provided by an untrained individual.[1] Describe the assist, cues, and specific technique(s) used. This can be difficult to do, especially when trying to be concise. Use knowledge of the intervention to describe what you are doing during the session to help the patient/client. A description of *how* your unique and sophisticated skills are used provides insight to the patient's need for skilled services and is a requirement for documentation. Also, in the initial documentation, include plans for skilled intervention that will be done (Examples 7-7 and 7-8).

Document why the intervention is medically necessary. The medical record should provide justification for the physical therapy intervention(s). This is a requirement in the initial documentation and progress notes and should be included anytime a new intervention is added. In addition, describe why the patient needs a particular intervention. Proving medical necessity can be difficult, but it is a requirement. Initially, the record should include any

---

Example 7-9. Five Scenarios Showing Medical Necessity for Intervention

1. Patient will receive passive stretching to increase joint ROM necessary for overhead activity.
2. Patient will receive gait and balance training to increase endurance and safety needed for independent household ambulation.
3. Patient will be educated on the proper use of the orthoses to protect healing tissues and prevent skin breakdown.
4. Patient will receive manual traction to remove pressure from nerve root and decrease pain.
5. Patient requires passive ROM performed by a therapist because of a new rotator cuff repair. The patient is unable to perform the treatment himself because of contralateral extremity ROM limitations.

Example 7-10. Third-Person Language

DO NOT WRITE:

I ambulated the client 50 feet and provided minimal assistance for balance and verbal cueing for upright posture because of postural sway.

Instead, emphasize the behavior performed by the patient.

The pt. ambulated 50 feet and required minimal assistance x 1 for balance and verbal cueing for upright posture because of postural sway and loss of balance.

TABLE 7-1

EXAMPLE OF ACTIVE AND PASSIVE RANGE OF MOTION DOCUMENTED IN A TABLE

		AROM (Degrees)	PROM (Degrees)
(R) Shoulder	Flexion	140	155
	Extension	10	15
	IR	50	55
	ER	45	55
(R) Elbow	Flexion	140	140
	Extension	−25	−20
	Supination	80	n/a
	Pronation	80	n/a

AROM = active range of motion; (L) = left; n/a = not applicable; PROM = passive range of motion; (R) = right; IR = internal rotation; ER = external rotation.

---

medical diagnosis or condition (including physical therapy diagnosis) that prevents the patient from performing the intervention independently. Next, one uses his or her scientific knowledge of the intervention and the condition and describes *why* the particular service will be provided. One may also include known evidence as a justification for a particular treatment (Example 7-9).

Documentation should be patient centered. Document using the *third person* because the emphasis is on what the patient can do or does (Example 7-10).

However, there are times when using the first person is unavoidable. This usually occurs after special situations and you are describing what happened in the narrative format. Documentation should never include references to the individual patient or client by his or her diagnosis (ie, the stroke patient).

Individual entries and the entire record should be organized. This applies to written medical records because the EMR provides an infrastructure for the organization of the record and individual entries. When writing notes by hand, use headings to group relevant information together, to indicate new sections, and to designate important patient information. Headings make the note easier to read and identify necessary information. Examples of appropriate section headings and subheadings can be found in Table 5-1. In instances in which there is a great deal of data that can easily become confusing to the reader, it is appropriate to use tables, columns, or lists. Tables are valuable when documenting range of motion or strength on several joints (Table 7-1).

Follow industry standards. Document according to widely accepted standards for writing in medical records. In handwritten documentation, write with black permanent ballpoint ink. Erasable ink or pencil should never be used. In handwritten records, avoid skipping lines in the record. Begin your note, starting with the date of service, on the line immediately below the prior entry. Do not skip lines in the middle of your notes. Skipping lines could allow someone to come back at a later date and fraudulently add in information. Include the patient's name and medical record number at minimum on new pages started in handwritten records.

> ## Example 7-11. Errors
>
> The pt. ~~ambulated~~ (MLE 1/17/19) transferred with minimal assist x 1 stabilizing the left knee to prevent buckling.

> ## Example 7-12. Multiple Pages
>
> "Continued next page. Sue Brooks, PT." Then, on the top of the next page, write "Continued from previous."

Avoid misuse of abbreviations. Use only industry-standard, facility-approved, medical terminology, symbols, and abbreviations (Appendix). It is important to also recognize that some facilities may prohibit all medical abbreviations due to the varied nature of their meanings. They can be misinterpreted and confusing, especially if a reader is unfamiliar with the abbreviations. When reading others' notes, realize some abbreviations have more than one meaning (eg, PT = physical therapist and prothrombin time). Read the entire note to determine the context of the abbreviation so that you can interpret it appropriately. Check with your facility regarding acceptable abbreviations and their use.

Writing late entries and addendums. If you must come back to a record later and document something that you have inadvertently omitted, then document the information as a *late entry* or *addendum*. A chart entry is considered a late entry when enough time has elapsed so that the date you are writing the late entry is different from the original documentation. In this case, the late entry should be placed in chronological order for the date that it is written and be identified as a late entry. Sign the late entry as you would any other documentation. If you immediately realize you have forgotten to write something that should have been included, write an addendum. An addendum is written immediately following the original documentation. Identify the additional information with the heading "Addendum:" following the original documentation without skipping a line. Sign the addendum as you would your original documentation. EMR systems will have specific directions for writing late entries and addendums or editing a note that has already been completed. Never rewrite or inappropriately add information to the original note.

Correcting errors. If you make an error while handwriting an entry into the medical record, correct it by placing a single straight line through the text. An individual reading the note should still be able to read the original text. Provide your initials and date next to the error (Example 7-11). Never use correction fluid or erasable ink in a medical record.

Using multiple pages. When handwritten documentation requires more than one page, make sure subsequent or additional pages include the patient's name, patient or chart number, and the date. Transition the information like shown in Example 7-12.

REVIEW QUESTIONS

1. How should a paper chart be stored once all documentation has been completed for a given date of service?
2. What types of documentation should be placed in the medical record that would help in making it complete?
3. Give an example of documenting a statement that is outside the physical therapist's scope of practice.
4. Describe "skilled" services and provide an example of how one should document the skills being provided to a patient.
5. True or false: Physical therapists should use as many abbreviations as possible.
6. True or false: It is good practice to make up abbreviations for a medical record.
7. What is meant by objective language?
8. How should one show the rationale for a treatment in the medical record?
9. What color ink should be used in handwritten notes?
10. How should errors be corrected?

APPLICATION EXERCISES

Consider which of the following entries would be inappropriate for documenting in a medical record, and indicate why:

1. The patient walked 50 feet.
2. The patient enjoys seeing her therapist 3 times per week.
3. AROM: (R) shoulder flexion 160 degrees; abduction 120 degrees.
4. The patient performed strengthening for the (R) LE.
5. The patient demonstrated excessive hip abduction with his prosthesis during ambulation.
6. Gait: the patient ambulated 100 feet ×2 with a hemi walker with minimal assist ×1 for advancing the (L) LE.
7. Bed mobility: patient rolls right and left independently, performs scooting and bridging independently, and requires min assist ×1 when coming to sit to support LE fracture.
8. HEP: instructed patient in a home program to be performed daily.

9. The patient complained of pain in the left knee limiting his ability to stand and ascend and descend stairs.

10. The patient is reporting improvement in his ankle range of motion as a result of the stretching completed in his home program.

Rewrite the following in a clear, concise manner so it would be acceptable for entry into a medical record.

11. The patient and the therapist walked 75 feet in the hallway one time with the therapist providing min assist to help the patient maintain her balance because of dizziness. The patient was using a front-wheeled walker.

12. The patient said that her pain was 3/10 on a pain scale. Following a manual muscle test, the patient's strength was 3/5 for the right biceps and 4/5 for the right triceps. The left biceps and triceps were both 5/5.

13. The patient demonstrated the following range of motion measurements: active range of motion for the right elbow was 140 degrees flexion and 10 degrees of hyperextension. Left active elbow range of motion was lacking 20 degrees from full extension and 90 degrees of flexion. Right knee active range of motion was 100 degrees flexion and lacking 10 degrees of extension. Left knee active range of motion was 0 degrees extension to 150 degrees flexion.

Identify the documentation errors in the following example:

Therapist: John Smith, PT

Physician: Dr. Harris

Date: November 7, 2019

Diagnosis: s/p (R) rotator cuff repair and acromioplasty

Next MD Appointment: November 14, 2019

Patient History: Patient fell on January 2, 2019, landing on the (R) UE. After fall, he complained of significant pain and sought medical attention. MRI revealed partial thickness tear of rotator cuff. The pt. reports he was placed in a sling for 2 weeks and then returned to work. Continued to have pain and dysfunction and recently underwent repair to (R) rotator cuff by Dr. Harris on November 1, 2019. Patient reports point tenderness along the spine of the scapula that is limiting him from performing his ADLs. Patient has not been sleeping well and reports pain at 8/10 on the pain scale. Patient has difficulty raising his arm overhead because of pain; however, pain decreases when arm is placed on his stomach.

Tests and Measures: AROM: flexion 30 degrees, abduction 90 degrees, IR 80 degrees, ER 15 degrees. PROM: flexion 60 degrees, abduction 100 degrees, IR 70 degrees, ER 20 degrees. Treatment included AROM and electrical stimulation using IFC and a quadrupolar electrode configuration with the frequency at 80 to 150 Hz for 20 minutes with ice.

Prognosis: s/p (R) rotator cuff repair and acromioplasty

Discharge Goals:

1. Independently perform ADLs within 6 to 8 weeks

2. Decrease complaints of pain to 0/10 within 6 to 8 weeks

3. Obtain functional ROM within 6 to 8 weeks

Interventions to Be Used: Modalities, ultrasound, electric stimulation, laser, manual therapy, PROM, stretching, and joint mobilizations. Therapeutic exercises and activities will be performed per protocol. The patient will be seen 2 to 3 times per week for 8 to 12 weeks.

REFERENCE

1. Hester H. Preparing for medical review: auditing your documentation. Paper presented at: Combined Sections Meeting of the American Physical Therapy Association. February 8-12, 2012; Chicago, IL.

CHAPTER 8

Documenting the Examination

Rebecca S. McKnight, PT, MS and Ralph R. Utzman, PT, MPH, PhD

CHAPTER OUTLINE

- Organizing the Information
- Documenting the Patient History
  - General Demographics
  - Current Condition(s) or Chief Complaint(s)
  - Activities and Participation
  - Clinical Tests
  - Medical/Surgical History
  - Medications
  - Growth and Development
  - Family History
  - Living Environment and Social History
  - Social/Health Habits and General Health Status
  - Formatting the History and Patient Interview Information
- Objective Data
  - Systems Review
  - Tests and Measures
  - Measuring Impairment
  - Measuring Function
    - Generic Versus Specific Measures
    - Patient Performance Versus Self-Report
  - Describing Interventions
  - Counting Minutes

Erickson ML, Utzman RR, McKnight RS.
Physical Therapy Documentation: From Examination to Outcome,
Third Edition (pp 69-80).
© 2020 Taylor & Francis Group.

CHAPTER OBJECTIVES

Upon completion of this chapter, the reader will be able to:

1. List sources of information for historical data
2. Differentiate between the Problem and Subjective sections of the note
3. Identify types of data that should be recorded in the Problem and Subjective sections of a SOAP note
4. Discuss how historical data inform the clinical decision-making process
5. When given information collected from a patient history, organize the information in logically sequenced Problem and Subjective sections
6. Identify types of data that should be recorded in the Objective section of the SOAP note
7. Discuss the purpose of the systems review
8. Discuss how objective data are used to inform the clinical decision-making process
9. Differentiate between measurements of impairments of body structure/function and measurements of functional activity limitations
10. Discuss characteristics of tests and measures (general vs specific and self-report vs performance based)
11. When provided data collected during a patient examination, arrange the data into a logically sequenced Objective section

KEY TERMS

examination
history
interview
objective
problem
reliability
skill
subjective
systems review
tests and measures
validity

KEY ABBREVIATIONS

FIM
Pr:
S:
SOAP

As described in Chapter 4, an episode of physical therapy care is initiated via the examination and evaluation process. Data gleaned during the examination via history taking, systems review, and tests and measures will be documented in an initial note. In this chapter, we consider the types of information and methods of documenting this information. The initial note will also include the therapist's interpretation of the data gleaned during the examination process. Specifics related to documenting the evaluation are described in Chapter 9.

A patient/client examination begins with the therapist gleaning a thorough history. During history taking, the therapist gathers information from the patient/client, family, other providers, and the medical record about the patient and his or her health condition, impairments, activities, and participation. This step is vital in identifying the patient's need for physical therapy services.[1,2] The history provides information that helps the therapist choose the appropriate tests and measures to perform as well as any modifications that may need to be made for standardized tests. The patient's goals, expectations, and educational needs are also identified.

ORGANIZING THE INFORMATION

If the Subjective, Objective, Assessment, and Plan (SOAP) note format is used, the examination information will be located in 3 distinct sections (Figure 8-1). The first section, called Problem (often abbreviated Pr:), contains information found in the medical record, physician referral, reports or results of laboratory tests, etc. The Problem section may be quite long if there is extensive information already available in the medical record. This is frequently the case in hospitals or other institutional settings. The second section is called Subjective (usually abbreviated S:) and contains information given by the patient, family, or caregiver.

"Subjective" refers to information that is gathered from a secondary source rather than from a direct measurement or observation. Subjective information is gathered during the patient interview and provides insight into what the patient knows about his or her condition and its impact on functional activities and participation.

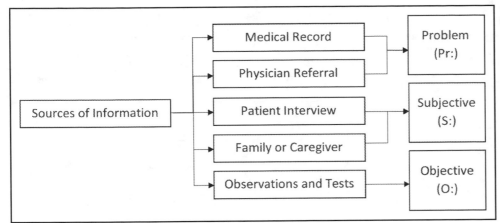

Figure 8-1. Organizing examination information in a SOAP note.

The third section is called Objective. Objective information is data gathered from direct observation or tests and measures. This information provides a clear picture of the patient's condition (including at a minimum impairments and functional limitations).

DOCUMENTING THE PATIENT HISTORY

Regardless of the documentation format used, it is helpful to identify where the history data originate from. This is essential if conflicting information is found. For example, a patient may indicate that he or she had a ruptured aorta, but upon review of his or her medical record, the physical therapist may find that the patient experienced a ruptured coronary artery. Recording both the information the patient provided as well as the information from the medical record can help demonstrate the patient's limited understanding of his or her condition.

When there is a significant amount of information to document related to the patient's history, it is helpful to organize the information into sections with subheadings. These subheadings allow for organization of the information presented so that specific data can be located more easily by the reader. The *Guide for Physical Therapist Practice*[3] describes several categories of historical data, which are summarized in Table 8-1. Any or all of these might appear in the Problem or Subjective section of the note depending on the source of information.

The subheadings used in each examination note will vary based on the patient's situation and the setting in which care is delivered. Some general guidelines of information to include in each subheading follow.

General Demographics

The initial note should include basic information about the patient's age, sex, and ethnicity. If the patient's primary language is not English, it should be noted here as well. If the patient has been referred to physical therapy by another provider, it is customary to include this information with the statement of the referral.

Current Condition(s) or Chief Complaint(s)

The physical therapist should document the patient's primary reason for seeking physical therapy or health care services. The patient's reason may be expressed as a symptom, such as pain, dizziness, etc, or in terms of activity limitations (eg, pain with lifting) or participation restrictions (eg, unable to work). The date of onset, mechanism of injury, and behavior of symptoms (location, duration, severity, and how symptoms change with activity) will provide important clues about the patient's problem and further guide the examination process. It is important to note what treatment has been provided for the patient so far and whether these treatments have helped. This portion of the patient interview should lead to a discussion of the patient's goals and expectations for physical therapy and set a foundation for the patient-therapist relationship.

Activities and Participation

The patient's level of activity and participation, both currently and before the injury/illness that brought him or her to physical therapy, should be determined. Information regarding the patient's functional status prior to the current situation typically comes from the patient; however, the information should be verified with a family member or caregiver when available. This information then will be compared with the objective information from the therapist's observations and function tests. It's important when obtaining information regarding the patient's prior level of function to not only ask about specific tasks the patient is or is not able to perform, but also it is helpful to ask the patient to describe a typical day and/or week. For example, a patient may indicate being independent with getting around the house, but when describing a typical day, the therapist may learn the patient spends most of the day in bed. Creating a

TABLE 8-1

CATEGORIES OF HISTORICAL DATA RECORDED IN A PHYSICAL THERAPY EXAMINATION

SUBHEADING	TYPE OF INFORMATION
General demographics	Age, education, primary language, race/ethnicity, sex
Activities and participation	Current and prior role functions (eg, self-care and domestic, education, work, community and social, and civic life)
Current condition(s)	Concerns that led the patient or client to seek the services of a physical therapist Current therapeutic interventions Mechanism of injury or disease, including date of onset and course of events Onset and pattern of symptoms Patient and family/caregiver goals and expectations Patient and family/caregiver perceptions and emotional response to current clinical situation Previous occurrence of current condition(s) Prior therapeutic interventions
Medications	Medications for current conditions Medications for other conditions Include prescription and over-the-counter medications and supplements
Other clinical tests	Laboratory and diagnostic tests Review of available records (medical/surgical) Review of other clinical findings
Medical/surgical history	Prior hospitalizations and surgeries Pre-existing medical and health conditions (comorbidities)
Growth and development	Developmental history Hand/foot dominance
Family history	Familial health risks
Living environment	Assistive technology Living environment and community characteristics Projected destination at conclusion of care
Social history	Cultural beliefs and behaviors Family/caregiver resources Social interactions and support systems
General health status	General health perceptions Mental functions (eg, memory, reasoning ability, depression, anxiety) Physical function (eg, mobility, sleep patterns, restricted bed days)
Social/health habits (past and current)	Behavioral health risks (eg, tobacco use, drug abuse) Level of physical fitness

Adapted from the American Physical Therapy Association. *Guide to Physical Therapist Practice.* 2016. http://guidetoptpractice.apta.org/. Accessed April 18, 2018 clear picture of the patient's prior level of function is important to help establish the need for physical therapy and to guide the remainder of the examination. Documenting good information about functional status will help determine which tests and measures should be performed later in the examination. In many cases, the expected outcome of therapy is to return the patient to his or her previous level of function, so documenting this information will be helpful in establishing a prognosis later in the note. The patient's current occupation and other social roles (student, mother, homemaker, retiree, etc.) should be documented. Documentation of the patient's work, school, home, and leisure activities provides important insight into the patient's prior level of function and contributes to setting goals for therapy. The physical therapist might also include information regarding prior occupations if this information has any bearing on the patient's current condition. For example, a patient may be retired from a job in the logging industry. The patient's previous work condition may have contributed to his or her current back problem.

Clinical Tests

The physical therapist should document pertinent medical tests and procedures that have been performed, such as clinical laboratory and radiology reports. Whenever possible, this information should be gathered from or confirmed by the medical record and documented in the physical therapy note. These reports give vital information about the patient's diagnosis, clinical medical condition, and precautions that may need to be followed. For instance, a patient with low hemoglobin and hematocrit levels may not tolerate physical activity, so the therapist may need to delay interventions until these levels return to normal.

Even though clinical test results may be available elsewhere in the patient's medical record, it is still important for the therapist to document them in his or her documentation to help support the therapist's clinical decision making. Test results contribute to the therapist's overall evaluation of the patient and often impact the physical therapy plan of care; if the therapist does not include this information in his or her documentation, the therapist's clinical thinking might be unclear. Also, documenting this information in the physical therapy note will allow the physical therapist assistant or others who are participating in or reviewing the physical therapy care of the patient to have ready access to the information. If the test result report is lengthy, it is acceptable for the therapist to summarize the key findings in the physical therapy note and refer readers to the full report (Example 8-1).

Medical/Surgical History

Many physical therapy patients have multiple medical conditions. These comorbidities may impact the patient's progress in therapy. For example, consider 2 patients who undergo knee replacement surgery. One patient has a

---

> ## Example 8-1. Documenting Results of Medical Tests
>
> <u>Clinical Tests:</u> Chest X-ray 11/14/2019 10:25 in the morning indicates atelectasis in the right lower lobe. Refer to radiology notes for further details.

---

history of asthma and requires a slightly longer course of therapy to build respiratory endurance after the surgery. The other patient has a history of diabetes and requires close monitoring of blood glucose levels during exercise. These patients' plans of care will need to take the comorbidities into account when considering intervention duration, parameters, and precautions. Whenever possible, this information should be gathered from or confirmed by the medical record. In settings where this is not possible, this information must be gathered through careful, thorough patient interviews.

Medications

The physical therapist should note every medication the patient is taking, including those for other health conditions. Besides helping alleviate the patient's symptoms or treating other health conditions, some medications may cause side effects or alter the patient's response to exercise or other activities. Be sure to include any over-the-counter medications and supplements the patient routinely uses.

Growth and Development

Physical therapists provide care for patients across the life span, and patients' activities and participation change with their life stages. Some patients access physical therapy to address developmental disabilities. In these cases, it is important to accurately document a thorough developmental history with special emphasis on participation and function in life tasks. This will help guide the selection of appropriate tests and measures for the objective portion of the examination.

Documentation of hand dominance is also important, especially in the case of upper extremity impairment. Treatment strategies and patient expectations may be different based on whether the injured extremity is dominant or nondominant.

Family History

Family health risks should be identified and documented as a mechanism for screening and prevention. For example, patients with a family history of heart disease, diabetes, stroke, or high blood pressure may need referral to a physician for further screening and intervention. For example, a 64-year-old woman is referred to physical therapy for evaluation of dizziness and balance problems. During the patient

---

Example 8-2A.
Stating the Problem

11/2/2019 PHYSICAL THERAPY INITIAL EVALUATION
PROBLEM

67-year-old woman s/p (R) THA referred 11/1/2019
for "Evaluate and Treat, partial weight-bearing (R)
LE" by Dr. David Jones.

Example 8-2B.
Stating the Problem

11/2/2019 PHYSICAL THERAPY INITIAL EVALUATION
PROBLEM

67-year-old woman

<u>Medical Diagnosis:</u> (R) THA, (R) lower lobe
pneumonia.

<u>Referral:</u> 11/1/2019 for "Evaluate and Treat, partial
weightbearing (R) LE" by Dr. David Jones.

<u>Clinical Tests:</u> chest X-ray 11/14/2019 10:25 AM indi-
cates atelectasis in the (R) lower lobe. Refer to radiology notes for further details.

---

interview, the therapist notes the patient's mother and grandfather both developed type 2 diabetes later in life. The patient reports that her dizziness is not affected by body position or head movement, and the therapist confirms this in her examination. The therapist refers the patient to her physician for further workup, who determines the patient does have diabetes.

Living Environment and Social History

In inpatient settings, physical therapists play a key role in discharge planning. They assess the patient's activity limitations and participation restrictions and make clinical judgments to predict the patient's functional status at discharge. As the patient prepares to go home, it is important to note the layout of the patient's home, the adaptive equipment the patient has available, and the support available to the patient at home or from the community. For patients in the outpatient setting, this information is also important to guide the treatment plan and optimize the patient's function in the home and community.

Physical therapists are expected to provide care that is culturally appropriate for the patient.[3] Along with the living environment, it is important to note the patient's health-related cultural beliefs, social interactions, and available support system.

Social/Health Habits and General Health Status

The goal of physical therapy is to maximize the patient's movement-related activity and optimize participation in his or her social roles. Patients' perceptions of their health can be impacted by physical, emotional, psychological, and social determinants. Discussing the patient's perception of his or her current and expected level of health should be a factor in determining the patient's goals for physical therapy.

Many health-related social habits can affect function and quality of life. It is important to note the patient's level of fitness, dietary habits, and use of substances such as tobacco and alcohol. A patient who engaged in regular physical activity before an illness or injury may tolerate a more aggressive exercise protocol than a patient who was previously sedentary. Patients who have poor dietary habits or who smoke may experience slower healing. Identifying these lifestyle habits can help guide goal setting, identify opportunities to improve physical fitness, and clarify needs for referrals for smoking cessation or dietary consultations.

Formatting the History and Patient Interview Information

The initial examination note should start with the time and date. It is customary to write the time using a 24-hour clock ("military time"); a regular 12-hour clock can be used as long as AM or PM is clearly indicated. If the note is handwritten in a record that includes multiple practitioners, a title is needed so that readers know what discipline the note is representing (eg, "Physical Therapy") and what type of note they are reading (eg, "Initial Evaluation Note"). In the case in which an interpreter is necessary to facilitate communication, it is important to document not only that an interpreter was used but also the relationship to the patient (if family or friend) or the name and organization the interpreter works for if a professional. Once these initial components are documented, the next thing to include is the first major heading (if using the SOAP format, the first major heading is "Problem" or Pr:). This heading should appear on the very next line below the date, time, and title. *Never* leave blank lines in handwritten notes.

When using the SOAP note format, the Problem section should include basic demographics of the patient, medical diagnosis, and referral information. This can be done in 1 or 2 narrative phrases (Example 8-2A).

Note that the passage includes the date of referral, the name of the physician, and a direct quote of the referral. If the patient has multiple diagnoses and/or a complex referral, subheadings can be used to separate the parts of this passage and then other information from the chart review following (Example 8-2B). Other headings that can be used would include reason for referral, patient's chief complaint, or primary diagnosis.

Example 8-3. Problem and Subjective

11/2/2019 10:45 PHYSICAL THERAPY EVALUATION NOTE
PROBLEM
24-year-old man referred by Dr. Jones 11/1/2019 0730 for "ROM exercises and gait training WBAT (L) LE. Pt. must wear Bledsoe brace while walking."
Diagnosis: ACL repair (L) knee yesterday.
Meds: Percocet prn. Last taken 2 hours ago.
SUBJECTIVE
HPI: Pt injured (L) knee 2 weeks ago while playing intramural flag football. Pt. was moving to avoid an opponent when he was struck on the LLE by another player. He was seen in the emergency room and referred to orthopedics. PMH: No previous surgeries.
C/C: Pt reports pain (L) knee. The pain increases with movement.

Living Environment/Social: The pt. lives in an upstairs apartment. He has 10 steps leading up to the apartment, with a handrail on the right going up. He has a roommate who can help with cooking and cleaning, but the pt. will need to be independent in ADLs.
Occupation: Pt. is a third-year physical therapy student.
Functional Status: Prior to injury, pt. was active in intramural sports. Since the injury, pt. has been using axillary crutches.
Pt. Goals: The pt. wishes to return to recreational sports. The pt. is scheduled to go on clinical internships next semester and will need to be independently mobile without assistive devices by mid-February.

Example 8-4. Documentation of Subjective Information from a Self-Referred Patient/Client

11/2/2019 14:30 PHYSICAL THERAPY EVALUATION NOTE
SUBJECTIVE
Chief Complaint: 55-year-old woman presents with complaints of vertigo.
HPI: Pt. experienced episode of severe vertigo 1 week ago when turning over in bed. The vertigo lasted for less than a minute and was accompanied by nausea and vomiting. She now reports feeling "off balance" and dizzy.
Symptoms are worse when she looks up, when she turns her head quickly, or when she bends over.
PMH: No previous surgeries. Pt. reports history of hypertension treated by Dr. Jennifer Jackson.

Medications: Captopril
Living Environment/Social: The patient lives in a 2-story home with her husband and daughter. There are 10 steps between levels with a handrail on the right side.
Occupation: Pt. is an accountant and plays golf weekly.
Functional Status: Prior to onset, pt. was independent in all mobility and ADLs. Since onset, she has been afraid to drive and is unable to golf. She notices that she holds onto walls and door frames when walking and feels unsteady when climbing stairs.
Pt. Goals: The patient wants to alleviate her symptoms, improve walking, and resume driving.

Next, the note should document information provided by the patient and/or the patient's family or caregivers. In the SOAP note, this begins with the new heading of "Subjective" (S:). As with the Problem section, information can be organized using subheadings as appropriate. Example 8-3 provides an example of the Problem and Subjective sections of an evaluation note for a patient in an acute care hospital.

Recall that the key difference between the Problem and Subjective sections is the source of the information. In Example 8-3, the patient's medications are documented in the beginning section, indicating the information was gleaned from the medical chart, as opposed to Example

8-4 in which the medication information was gleaned from the patient and therefore documented in the Subjective section of the note.

OBJECTIVE DATA

Once the physical therapist has documented the patient's history information gathered through a review of the medical record and patient/caregiver interviews, the physical therapist will initiate the physical examination. The physical examination consists of a systems review and specific tests and measures essential to determine the patient's

> # Example 8-5. Documenting the Systems Review
>
> Systems Review:
> Cardiovascular/Pulmonary: HR, 80; BP, 110/70; RR, 16; no edema present; Integumentary: Skin color and texture are unimpaired; Musculoskeletal: Gross strength and ROM (B) UE, (R) LE unimpaired. Impaired strength and ROM (L) LE, see below. Neuromuscular: Neurovascular structures are intact; Communication/Cognition: Pt. alert & oriented x 4. Pt. wears hearing aid. Note: References to "see below" refer the reader to additional test(s) or measure(s) that were performed as well as the result(s).

physical therapy diagnosis and to guide the development of the plan of care. Although information gathered from the patient and/or caregiver often contains information that communicates their perspective and can be subjective in nature, data and information from the physical examination should be based on things that can be observed or measured. These observations and measurements are generally presented in this section without judgments or evaluation; analysis of the data occurs in a later section of the note. In addition to data from the physical examination, if any interventions are provided, they will be documented in this section of the note as well. In a SOAP note, this section will be labeled as the Objective section and will include subheadings including the systems review, tests and measures, and interventions (if provided). If interventions are provided, they should be presented as well. As with the Subjective sections, the use of further subheadings can help to emphasize important information and to make specific facts easier for readers to find.

Systems Review

The systems review is defined by the *Guide to Physical Therapist Practice*[3] as a "brief or limited examination" that includes screening various body systems for anatomical or physiological impairments. The purpose of the systems review is to establish, along with data from the chart review and patient interview, the need for the physical therapy examination and to guide the physical therapist's selection of more specific tests and measures.[3] In addition, as primary care providers, it is important that physical therapists screen patients for common conditions that might require referral to a physician such as hypertension or skin cancer. The systems review should be brief, but, at a minimum, it should include screenings of the cardiovascular, integumentary, musculoskeletal, and neuromuscular systems along with the patient's cognitive status, communication abilities, and affect. If the physical therapist finds no impairments in a particular system, the therapist simply notes "unimpaired" under the appropriate subheading. The specific screening(s) and result(s) that lead to this clinical decision should be documented. If evidence of impairment is found, the findings are briefly noted or summarized, and the reader is referred to the tests and measures section for further details. An example of the systems review is provided in Example 8-5.

Tests and Measures

The tests and measures portion of the note provides results of specific tests performed by the therapist designed to determine the impairment and functional limitations that will be addressed by physical therapy. The physical therapist selects tests and measures based on the information collected from the chart review, patient interview, and systems review.[3] Thorough and accurate documentation of tests and measures provides baseline data about the patient's impairments, activity limitations, and participation restrictions. This baseline serves as the starting point for developing a patient prognosis and plan of care and demonstrating patient improvement over time. Selecting appropriate tests and measures involves deciding what aspects of "health" need to be measured and then matching measurement tools appropriately. Physical therapists should have adequate background knowledge of the measurement properties associated with tests and measures, including reliability (test-retest and inter-rater), validity, responsiveness, and the test's ability to measure change. A listing of categories and general tests and measures used by physical therapists can be found in the *Guide to Physical Therapist Practice*[3]; specific tests and measures are described on the American Physical Therapy Association's PT Now site (www.PTNow.org).

Measuring Impairment

The physical therapist should consider identifying impairments important to the patient population and determine appropriate tools to measure the impairments. For example, a physical therapist will need to examine range of shoulder motion in individuals with adhesive capsulitis and will therefore use goniometric measurements as an appropriate outcome measure. On the other hand, consider a patient with lateral epicondylitis. These patients rarely have limited range of motion, so goniometric measurements may not be appropriate. It may be more appropriate to measure pain during gripping or lifting tasks. Other impairments often measured include strength, sensation, endurance, reflexes, and balance.

Measuring Function

Generic Versus Specific Measures

Finch et al[4] described the use of both generic and specific tools for measuring function. Generic measures, or general health status questionnaires, are not specific to any one pathology or diagnosis. Generic measures, such as the Functional Independence Measure (FIM),[5] are used to assess "overall" aspects of the individual's functional capacity, such as walking, transferring, bathing, and dressing. Generic measures are appropriate for both healthy and unhealthy populations and allow clinicians to assess physical function alone or physical function combined with societal integration.[4] Some generic measures are also used to evaluate emotional response(s) to injury and psychosocial issues through subscales. In addition to the FIM, other popular generic measurement tools include the 36-item Short-Form Health Survey,[6] its shortened counterpart the 12-item Short-Form Health Survey,[7] and the Sickness Impact Profile.[8]

Specific measures of function include pathology (disease)-specific, body part (body region)–specific, and patient-specific measures. Pathology-specific measurement tools include items that are geared specifically to assess function and disability for individuals with a given pathology, such as the Arthritis Impact Measurement Scales[9] and the Fibromyalgia Impact Questionnaire.[10] In body part—or region-specific tools, such as the Disabilities of the Arm, Shoulder, and Hand Questionnaire,[11] the Neck Disability Index,[12] and the Oswestry Low Back Pain Questionnaire,[13] patients are scored based on a set of predetermined tasks using the involved body part (eg, writing or turning a key on the Disabilities of the Arm, Shoulder, and Hand Questionnaire). Patient-specific measurement tools allow each patient to identify his or her own set of functional tasks he or she may be unable to perform because of the injury or illness. In using a patient-specific measure, the patient is not provided with a predetermined list of functional tasks. For example, the Patient-Specific Functional Scale[14] requires the provider to ask the patient to identify 3 to 5 important activities that he or she is having difficulty with or is unable to perform because of the illness or injury. Then, the patient is asked to rate the level of difficulty on a scale of 0 to 10, with 0 indicating "unable to perform" and 10 being "able to perform at preinjury level."[14]

Authors have identified strengths and weaknesses of both generic and specific measurement tools. First, generic health measures allow comparisons to be made across different patient cohorts and have relatively "good measurement properties."[4(p17)] Nevertheless, generic measures may hide or mask functional problems specific to certain pathologies. Some patients seen in an outpatient orthopedic setting may score very high on generic health measures. For example, the patient with lateral epicondylitis could obtain a perfect score on the FIM yet be unable to work because of pain and pain-induced weakness. Generic or general health measurement tools may also be "less sensitive to change than more specific measures"[4(p17)] and may "hide sensitive clinical changes."[15(p1)] In these cases, the instrument does not capture relevant patient changes because of interventions.

Strengths of specific measurement tools have been identified. Specific tools measure functional problems often unique to a pathology or body part and thus "capture" specific problems for that population. Questions are targeted at identifying disability due to a specific pathology, or injury to a body part, rather than evaluating general health-related quality of life. More specific functional tasks that appear on these types of questionnaires are generally not included in a generic tool. In addition, functional changes occurring as a result of an intervention may be seen more clearly using a specific tool rather than a generic quality of life questionnaire. However, weaknesses of specific tools have been described by Finch et al.[4] These authors reported that the comparison of scores on specific tools is limited to patients with the same condition or problem of the same body part (eg, patients with rotator cuff syndrome or patients with acute low back pain). Finally, a specific measure may not capture general quality of life changes.[4]

Patient Performance Versus Self-Report

In performance-based outcome measures, the patient is required to perform a set of functional tasks, such as the FIM. In using the FIM, the patient is assessed according to his or her ability to (1) perform self-care skills (eg, feeding and dressing); (2) control bowel/bladder function; (3) transfer; (4) move (eg, gait and stair climbing); (5) communicate; and (6) interact socially, including memory and problem solving.

Function and disability assessments can also rely on "self-report." In self-report measures, the patient completes a questionnaire, rating his or her overall performance on a predetermined set of functional tasks. An example of a patient self-reported functional measure is the Oswestry Low Back Pain Questionnaire, which is often used to assess the functional status of patients with back pain. Other examples of self-reported questionnaires include the 36-item Short-Form Health Survey, the Neck Disability Index, and the Patient-Rated Wrist Evaluation.[16]

Describing Interventions

Patient care activities include both direct patient interventions as well as communication and coordination with other health care providers. It is essential that documentation clearly describes how the patient's physical care has been coordinated with other members of the health care team. The importance of recording this documentation was covered previously in Chapter 3. Some examples are provided in Examples 8-2A and 8-2B.

Similarly, document any instructions that have been given. This includes discussions of informed consent (see Chapter 3) regarding the planned interventions with the patient. Do not forget to document instructions given to family members or other caregivers. Besides documenting what instructions were given, provide details on the teaching methods used and the patient's (or caregiver's) response

Example 8-6. Documenting Instructions and Informed Consent

Discussed purposes and procedures for selective wound debridement, as well as risk of bleeding or infection. Discussed use of sterile technique to reduce these risks. Discussed alternatives (whirlpool, wet-to-dry dressings) that will require more frequent therapy and carry similar risks. Pt. was given the opportunity to ask questions before giving consent to the procedure.

Instructed pt. in prone-on-elbows positioning 30 seconds x 5 reps, 3 times daily. Pt. was able to demonstrate this exercise correctly without verbal cues.

Taught the pt.'s husband techniques for guarding the pt. during home balance exercises. After a demonstration of proper body position and hand placement, pt.'s husband was able to safely guard the pt.

Example 8-7. Documenting Objective Information

Systems Review:

Cardiovascular/Pulmonary: HR, 80; BP, 110/70; RR, 16

Integumentary: Skin is intact, no abnormalities observed, (-) edema.

Musculoskeletal: Gross strength and ROM (B) UE, (R) LE unimpaired. Impaired strength and ROM (L) LE, see below.

Neuromuscular: Sensation is intact to light touch.

Communication/Cognition: Pt. alert & oriented x 4. Pt. wears hearing aid.

Functional Status: Sit-stand with minimal assistance of 1 for initiation of forward trunk movement and hip extension. Ambulates 10 feet per 30 seconds with walker, min A of 1 for advancement of walker and to maintain TDWB LLE. After ambulation, HR, 106; BP, 128/76; RR, 22.

AROM: (L) knee flexion 5-75°, hip flexion 0-95°.

Strength: (L) hip flexors and knee extensors 3+/5, (L) ankle plantarflexion and dorsiflexion 4+/5.

Today's Treatment: Gait and transfer training as described above for 15 minutes. Therapeutic exercise for a total of 20 minutes, including AROM (L) hip & knee flexion 10 reps, cued pt. to hold movement at maximum hip/knee flexion for 5 seconds with each repetition. Instructed Pt. in supine (L) straight leg raises 3 sets of 10 reps. Pt. was instructed to perform these exercises in his room later this afternoon. Pt. was able to demonstrate each exercise correctly.

to the instruction. Some examples are provided in Example 8-6.

Document all interventions and describe all parameters associated with the treatment. For example, when describing an exercise session, the therapist documents the type of equipment used, the joint(s) and movement(s) involved, the mode (active, passive, or resisted), the level of resistance, the number of repetitions and sets, and the length of rest periods between exercises. For patients with cardiovascular impairments or poor endurance, the documentation of vital signs before, during, and after exercise is warranted. When documenting the use of physical and electrotherapeutic agents, include the type of modality and all of the parameters (waveform, duration, temperature, frequency, intensity, etc) of the modality (Example 8-7).

When documenting interventions, the therapist should demonstrate the skill required to perform the treatment provided. In order to be reimbursed, the documentation must prove the treatment provided required decision-making capacity and the unique skills of a qualified provider. If such skill is not accurately described, the reader might assume that the patient could have completed the task or exercise without help or that a family member or other health care worker could have provided the assistance with less cost (see Example 8-8).

Counting Minutes

Medicare, insurance companies, and other third-party payers are reviewing therapists' documentation and billing with increasing scrutiny. They often compare the bills submitted with care documentation to look for fraud and

abuse. If a clear relationship cannot be made between the care documented and the services billed, the payer may deny the claim. In most care settings, physical therapists are required to document the number of actual minutes spent on each type of activity or treatment performed with each patient. This can be accomplished by noting the number of minutes spent on various activities in the Objective section.

REVIEW QUESTIONS

1. Describe the types of historical information that should be documented in the medical record.

2. What are the sources of information in the Problem (Pr:) and Subjective (S:) sections of a note?

3. Discuss the relationship between historical data and the tests and measures portion of the examination.

4. Outline an appropriate structure for the Problem and Subjective sections of a note documenting an initial patient encounter/evaluation.

5. List the information found within the Assessment and Plan sections of the SOAP note.

6. Describe the relationship between the examination and the evaluation.

7. How should the physical therapist construct a physical therapy diagnosis?

8. List considerations for developing a prognosis.

9. List and describe the components of a well-written goal.

10. How can a physical therapist integrate evidence regarding tests and measure into goal statements?

11. How does the physical therapist assistant use the information documented in the Assessment and Plan section of a SOAP note? How can the therapist structure the note to enhance the physical therapist/physical therapist assistant relationship?

12. Outline an appropriate structure for the documentation of the Assessment and Plan sections of a SOAP note.

APPLICATION EXERCISES

1. Provide the subheading for each of the following types of subjective data:
   a. Symptoms, such as pain
   b. Age
   c. Number of steps to get into the patient's home
   d. Type of surgery performed
   e. Patient's ability to get in/out of bed
   f. Ability to ambulate before surgery
   g. Work tasks
   h. Reports of seeking care from a chiropractor
   i. Patient's prior health status
   j. Hand dominance
   k. Patient's mother died of a stroke
   l. Results of blood work

2. For each of the examples in Exercise 1, how would you determine whether the information should be documented in the Problem or Subjective section of the note? Which source do you think would be best for each item?

3. Write each of the following in a clear, concise manner:
   a. The patient told you that her pain was a 6 on a 0 to 10 scale.
   b. The patient told you she feels dizzy when shopping; dizziness is the worst when walking down the aisle of a supermarket.

Example 8-8.
Skilled Versus Unskilled Language

Unskilled language: "The pt. ambulated with a walker for 20 feet, PWB LLE, with minimal assistance."

Skilled language: "The pt. ambulated with a walker for 20 feet, PWB LLE. The pt. required minimal assistance for walker placement, tactile cues to maintain PWB LLE, and instruction on proper gait sequence." The therapist was providing ongoing assessment, education, and cues for safety that require the skills and judgment of a physical therapist.

---

c. The patient's husband told you that his wife has fallen at home several times. They had to call an ambulance to get her up off the floor.

d. The patient told you that she gets tired and short of breath when vacuuming, cleaning the bathroom, and doing other household tasks.

e. The patient told you that she lives alone. She has neighbors and friends from church who stop by. Her daughter, who lives in another state, calls her 2 to 3 times per week.

4. Review the Problem and Subjective sections of the following note written about a patient seen in an outpatient clinic. Is any critical information missing? Does the note include information about activity limitations and participation restrictions? What questions would the physical therapist ask to gain missing information? What is the best source for this information?

11/30/2019 14:30 PHYSICAL THERAPY EVALUATION NOTE

PROBLEM

24 y.o. man referred by Dr. Tracy Frum for "Evaluate and treat"

Diagnosis: Low back pain

SUBJECTIVE

C/C: Pt. reports pain in the right lower back and buttock

HPI: Patient injured at work 2 weeks ago while lifting boxes

PMH: Tonsillectomy in 1994

Living Environment/Social: The patient lives in an apartment with 2 roommates.

Occupation: Patient is a graduate student. He has a part-time job with UPS.

Pt. Goals: Reduce back pain

5. Review the list of tests and measures in the Guide to Physical Therapist Practice. Choose one category and identify one test/measure that can be used to collect data for that category. Does the test provide information

regarding impairments or function? Is it a self-report measure or a performance measure? Research the reliability and validity of the test/measure you selected.

6. Write the following statements in a more clear and concise manner as it would appear in the medical record.

   a. The patient had trouble standing up from a seated position. The therapist applied tactile and verbal cues for the patient to lean forward and push up with her hands and provided minimal assist for balance on initial standing.

   b. The patient's active range of motion for right shoulder abduction was from 0 degrees to 80 degrees; the patient reported pain at end range.

   c. During the systems review, the measurements taken for blood pressure were 130/90, heart rate 98 bpm, oxygen saturation was 98%, and respiratory rate was 12 breaths/minute.

7. While examining a patient who has been experiencing falls, the following information was collected. Organize the information into a concise Objective section.

Patient's blood pressure is 128/78 and her heart rate is 72 bpm. She has an abrasion on her forehead slightly to the left of midline. She walks with slow steps and a wide base of support, holding onto walls and doorways for support. The only gross active range of motion impairments you notice is a limitation in shoulder flexion bilaterally, and gross strength is symmetrical. The patient is alert and oriented and follows instructions accurately. She wears bifocal glasses. The following tests and measures were performed during the examination. The patient's gait speed is 0.6 m/s. She scores 16/24 on the Dynamic Gait Index. Static standing balance on firm surface with arms crossed and feet together, she can stand for 30 seconds without assistance; the same position with eyes closed elicits backward trunk sway after 12 seconds. On a foam surface with arms crossed and feet together, she exhibits posterior trunk sway after 18 seconds; with her eyes closed standing on foam, she loses her balance after 5 seconds and needs assist to avoid a fall. She scores 42 out of 56 possible points on the Berg Balance Scale. Deep tendon reflexes are 2+ throughout. Sensation to light touch is normal using monofilament testing. No nystagmus is noted with movement or at rest. Active range of motion of right shoulder flexion is limited to 0 to 125 degrees and the left to 0 to 115 degrees. Passive range of motion of right shoulder flexion is 0 to 130 degrees and left 0 to 120 degrees with capsular end feel. Quadriceps strength and hip abductor strength are 4/5 bilaterally via manual muscle test.

REFERENCES

1. Quinn L, Gordon J. *Functional Outcomes Documentation for Rehabilitation.* St. Louis, MO: Saunders; 2003.

2. Stewart D, Abeln S. *Documenting Functional Outcomes in Physical Therapy.* St. Louis, MO: Mosby-Year Book; 1993.

3. American Physical Therapy Association. *Guide to Physical Therapist Practice.* 2016. http://guidetoptpractice.apta.org/. Accessed April 18, 2018.

4. Finch E, Brooks D, Stratford P, Mayo N. *Physical Rehabilitation Outcome Measures.* 2nd ed. Philadelphia, PA: Lippincott Williams and Wilkins; 2002.

5. Uniform Data System for Medical Rehabilitation. About the FIM system. http://www.udsmr.org. Accessed May 3, 2019.

6. Ware JJ, Snow K, Kosinski M, Gandek B. *SF-36 Health Survey Manual and Interpetation Guide.* Boston, MA: The Health Institute, New England Medical Center; 1993.

7. Ware JJ, Kosinski M, Keller S. A 12-item short form health survey: construction of scales and preliminary tests of reliability and validity. *Med Care.* 1996;34:220-233.

8. Bergner M, Bobbitt R, Carter W, Gilson B. The Sickness Impact Profile: development and final revision of a health status measure. *Med Care.* 1981;19:788-805.

9. Rhumatology ACo. Arthritis Impact Measurement Scales (AIMS). https://www.rheumatology.org/I-Am-A/Rheumatologist/Research/Clinician-Researchers/Arthritis-Impact-Measurement-Scales-AIMS. Published 2019. Accessed May 3, 2019.

10. American College of Rheumatology. Fibromyalgia Impact Questionnaire (FIQ). https://www.rheumatology.org/I-Am-A/Rheumatologist/Research/Clinician-Researchers/Fibromyalgia-Impact-Questionnaire-FIQ. Published 2019. Accessed May 3, 2019.

11. Gummesson C, Atroshi I, Ekdahl C. The disabilities of the arm, shoulder and hand (DASH) outcome questionnaire: longitudinal construct validity and measuring self-rated health change after surgery. *BMC Musculoskelet Disord.* 2003;4:11.

12. Vernon H, Mior S. Neck Disability Index: a study of reliability and validity. *J Manipulative Physiol Ther.* 1991;14:409-415.

13. Fairbank J, Pynsent P. The Owestry Disability Index. *Spine.* 2000;25:2940-2952.

14. Westaway M, Stratfor P, Binkley J. The patient specific functional scale: validation of its use in persons with neck dysfunction. *J Orthop Sports Phys Ther.* 1998;27:331-338.

15. Hart D. What should you expect from the study of clinical outcomes? *J Orthop Sports Phys Ther.* 1998;28:1-2.

16. MacDermid J, Tottenham V. Responsiveness of the disability of the arm, shoulder and hand (DASH) and patient-related wrist/hand evaluation (PRWHE) in evaluating change after hand therapy. *J Hand Ther.* 2004;17:18-23.

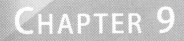

CHAPTER 9

Documenting the Evaluation

Rebecca S. McKnight, PT, MS and Mia L. Erickson, PT, EdD

CHAPTER OUTLINE

Erickson ML, Utzman RR, McKnight RS.
Physical Therapy Documentation: From Examination to Outcome,
Third Edition (pp 81-96).
© 2020 Taylor & Francis Group.

CHAPTER OBJECTIVES

Upon completion of this chapter, the reader will be able to:

1. Outline the information recorded in the Assessment and Plan sections of a SOAP note
2. Describe the relationship between the evaluation and the examination
3. Integrate a physical therapy diagnosis into the documentation
4. Discuss the use of "rehabilitation potential" in clinical documentation
5. Integrate comorbidities, complications, and complexities into the clinical documentation
6. Describe the clinical decision-making process used in establishing a patient prognosis
7. Construct short- and long-term goals in the form of behavioral objectives that include all pertinent information
8. Integrate scientific evidence on tests and measures into a goal
9. Organize given information into a properly structured assessment and plan

KEY TERMS

assessment
discharge goal
expected outcome
long-term goal
outcome
physical therapy diagnosis
plan
plan of care
problem list
prognosis
short-term goal
skilled services

KEY ABBREVIATIONS

A:
DASH
LTG
P:
SOAP
STG

Throughout the examination, the physical therapist interprets the findings from the history, systems review, and tests and measures. This is the initial stage of the physical therapist's evaluation. At the conclusion of the interviews and physical examination, the physical therapist synthesizes the information to determine the physical therapy diagnosis, prognosis, and plan of care. Although it may seem that the examination and evaluation processes are linear in nature (ie, the examination points to the evaluation, which then leads to the diagnosis, prognosis, and plan of care) (Figure 9-1), in reality there is a dynamic interplay that occurs throughout the initial patient encounter. Throughout the examination, the physical therapist makes

clinical judgments on various pieces of subjective and objective data. Depending on the data, the physical therapist probes further or moves on in a different direction. This is somewhat of a step forward–step back approach, allowing the therapist to rule in and rule out various impairments, activity limitations, and participation restrictions. Jones[1] described this clinical reasoning process as "cyclic" and used the "hypothetico-deductive method" to describe the decision-making process used during a physical therapy examination. Using this strategy, during the examination and evaluation processes, the physical therapist develops an initial hypothesis of the clinical problem(s) and proceeds with the examination by choosing questions, tests, or measures that confirm or deny the working hypothesis. Each question or test will provide information that will feed back into the process until sufficient information is obtained to make a clinical decision about the patient and the intervention plan.[1] The physical therapist documents these clinical judgments and decisions within the Assessment and Plan sections of the Subjective, Objective, Assessment, and Plan (SOAP) note.

DOCUMENTING THE EVALUATION INCLUDING THE PLAN OF CARE

Collectively, the Assessment (A:) and Plan (P:) are often referred to as the plan of care, or treatment plan. Some third-party payers, or insurers, have specific guidelines for information included in a plan of care,[2] and it is the physical therapist's responsibility to stay abreast of documentation guidelines and requirements for care plans because documentation requirements change frequently and vary across states, payers, and settings. A template for creating a plan of care can be found in Figure 9-2 and can be used when learning this aspect of documentation. This template provides components of the A: and P: sections of the initial documentation; however, many variations exist, and different facilities may have different policies for placement

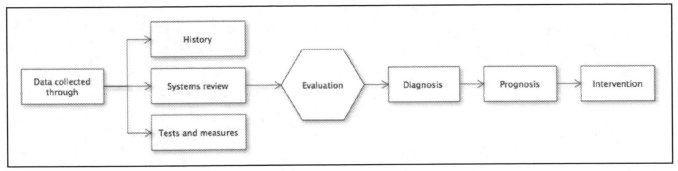

Figure 9-1. Linear view of clinical decision making in physical therapy.

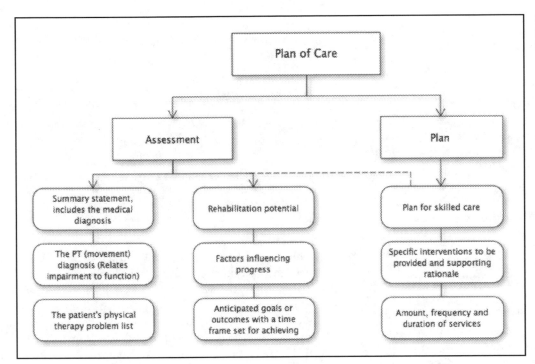

Figure 9-2. Template for the initial Assessment and Plan (plan of care).

of information within the initial documentation. Once the necessary components have been learned, one can be flexible in the arrangement and placement within the documentation to comply with various facility, or even payer, policies. In addition, the authors of the text chose to organize the contents using the SOAP structure but realize that in the clinical setting these sections may be written as one document called the plan of care. As stated previously, the emphasis should be on the contents and quality of documentation.

The Assessment and Plan are often the most difficult sections of the note to write. It is the physical therapist's chance to articulate and summarize the reason for the intervention plan, realizing others (eg, physical therapist assistants and third-party payers) will be reading the plan of care to aid in their decision making regarding the patient. In the Assessment section, the physical therapist assigns clinical meaning, or value, to the data collected during the examination process, and in the Plan section, the therapist describes what he or she plans to do to help with the patient's problems. All information documented

in this section of the note is substantiated by data collected in the examination and documented in the Subjective and Objective sections. To construct the Assessment and Plan, sentences, paragraphs, and lists are used to give a clear picture of the therapist's impression of the patient and "tell the patient's story." The plan of care should include a summary statement, the physical therapy diagnosis, a physical therapy problem list, a prognosis statement, patient goals, and planned interventions.

Summary Statement, Diagnosis, and Problem List

Summary Statement

The evaluation should include a patient summary. This consists of a brief statement, or set of statements, that describe the patient (ie, age, sex, and medical diagnosis). It answers the questions "Who is this patient?" and "What is wrong with him or her?" The summary often includes a patient's medical diagnosis. The medical diagnosis comes

Example 9-1. Physical Therapy Summary Statements

A: 69-year-old female admitted 2 days ago after fall down stairs sustaining a (R) femur fracture; now 1 day status postpinning.

A: 8-year-old female with myelomeningocele at the L1-2 level status post-recent growth spurt and functional decline.

A: 17-year-old female 2 weeks status post-right bimalleolar fracture.

Example 9-2. Physical Therapy Diagnoses

A: 69-year-old woman admitted 2 days ago after fall down stairs sustaining a right femur fracture; now 1 day status postpinning. Physical Therapy Diagnosis: Decreased ROM, strength, and weight bearing limiting the pt.'s ability to ambulate, transfer, and return to independent living, self-care, driving, and home-management tasks.

A: 8-year-old girl with myelomeningocele at the L1-2 level status post-recent growth spurt and functional decline. Physical Therapy Diagnosis: Impaired strength and sensation limiting pt.'s ability to ambulate independently in the home, school, or community and perform independent self-care and transfers; puts pt. at risk for skin breakdown.

A: 17-year-old girl 2 weeks status post-right bimalleolar fracture. Physical Therapy Diagnosis: Impaired ROM and strength associated with fracture limiting independent home, school, and community ambulation, driving, and participation in recreational activities.

from the patient's referral, the medical record, or even from the patient. The medical diagnosis is often the patient's pathology, disease, injury, or illness, such as multiple sclerosis, spinal cord injury, or humerus fracture. It may also include the relevant *International Classification of Diseases, Tenth Revision* code(s) (Example 9-1).

Physical Therapy Diagnosis

This section should also include a physical therapy diagnosis. This is a diagnosis of the patient's movement disorders or dysfunction, and it describes the impact of an injury or condition on function at the systems level (especially the movement system) and at the whole-person level.[3] The physical therapist uses a diagnosis process that includes integrating and explaining relevant data obtained during the examination and describing the patient/client condition in terms that will guide the prognosis and interventions.[3] The diagnostic "label" indicates the primary dysfunction to be addressed by the physical therapy interventions.[3] To document the physical therapy diagnosis, provide a statement(s) describing the relationship between the patient's impairments (identified in the examination data) and his or her activity limitations and participation restrictions (movement dysfunction). Also, document potential disabilities that may result if the impairments and functional deficits are not addressed appropriately. Use an appropriate heading (eg, physical therapist diagnosis or movement dysfunction) when documenting the physical therapy diagnosis so it is not confused with the medical diagnosis. Additional examples of documenting a physical therapy diagnosis can be found in Chapter 4.

In Example 9-2, note how the impairments (decreased range of motion, strength, and mobility), all identified on the examination, have been linked to the patient's specific functional problems (ambulation, transfers, return to independent living, etc).

Physical Therapy Problem List

In this section, the physical therapist provides a list of specific physical therapy problems that will be addressed

with the intervention. A problem list often includes some impairments, but most problems should focus on patient-specific activity limitations and participation restrictions identified during the examination. To create the problem list, the therapist reviews the examination data and identifies relevant patient complaints and functional deficits revealed during the patient/caregiver interviews as well as abnormal results from tests and measures identified in the examination and records them in a list format. The problem list adds more detailed information to the physical therapy diagnosis, and it serves as a framework to create the latter components of the plan of care (Example 9-3).

There may be times when the therapist chooses to integrate the physical therapy diagnosis and the problems list. In doing so, the problems are listed in a manner that relates a specific impairment to a specific activity limitation or participation restriction. One benefit of this is that it maintains the focus of the problem list on patient-specific function (Example 9-4).

THE PATIENT'S PROGNOSIS

A statement of the patient's prognosis should also be included. There are 3 components to the prognosis: (1) a statement regarding the patient's potential to benefit from the rehabilitation program, (2) a statement regarding problems or issues that may influence the intervention or the progress, and (3) a list of outcome goals showing the

Example 9-3. Physical Therapy Diagnosis and Problem List in Sequential Form

A: 69-year-old woman admitted 2 days ago after fall down stairs sustaining a (R) femur fracture; now 1 day status postpinning. Physical Therapy Diagnosis: Decreased ROM, strength, and weight bearing limiting the pt.'s ability to ambulate, transfer, and return to independent living, self-care, driving, and home-management tasks. Problem List: (1) Decreased hip and knee active ROM; (2) decreased strength in the (R) lower extremity; (3) decreased ability to bear weight in the (R) LE causing impaired balance; (4) dependent with bed and chair transfers; (5) dependent with sit-to-stand; (6) unable to ambulate without assistance; (7) unable to ascend and descend stairs; and (8) unable to perform independent self-care, home-management, or drive.

Example 9-4. Physical Therapy Diagnosis and Problem List in Integrated Form

A: 8-year-old girl with myelomeningocele at the L1-2 level status post-recent growth spurt and functional decline. Physical Therapy Diagnosis and Problem List: (1) Impaired motor function limiting the pt.'s ability to independently ambulate in her home, school, or community; (2) impaired motor function limiting pt.'s ability to perform independent self-care and transfers; and (3) impaired sensory integrity making pt. at risk for skin breakdown.

"intended results" of the physical therapy interventions. Goals also include a specific target date for when they will be achieved.

Rehabilitation Potential

In many cases, the physical therapist uses the terms *excellent*, *good*, *fair*, or *poor* to document a patient's rehabilitation potential. Although documenting potential in this manner is fairly common in clinical practice, there are no well-established criteria that constitute excellent, good, fair, or poor potential. In addition, authors have shown this method is not reliable between different therapists.[4] When using this terminology to describe rehabilitation potential, it seems if the physical therapist has considered all the necessary factors and set appropriate goals and time frames, then the patient's potential to meet the established

Example 9-5. Rehabilitation Potential

1. The pt.'s potential to benefit from therapy and achieve the goals stated is excellent because of his excellent motivation and health status.
2. The pt.'s potential to benefit from the intervention is good. Time since injury may influence how quickly the pt. may recover.
3. The pt. has good potential to achieve the goals established; however, his medical history, including diabetes and congestive heart failure, may influence length of recovery.
4. The pt. has good potential to achieve the established goals; however, chronic wound on the sound limb will interfere with gait training.

goals should be good. If the potential is poor, then the therapist should reconsider whether the patient is appropriate for therapy services or reconsider the established goals. Although the outcomes statements (patient goals) indicate in detail what the expected prognosis is, providing a general statement of potential can be helpful in communicating an overall prognosis. For example, "the patient should be able to return to full function" or, alternatively, "it is unlikely the patient will be able to safely return to his or her current working environment." This avoids general statements like "excellent potential for recovery" and rather speaks to broad but specific functional expectations.

Factors That May Influence the Intervention, Progress, or Outcome

It is imperative that the therapist documents any issues that might influence the intervention plan and recovery time. These issues may include (1) comorbidities, or concomitant diagnoses unrelated to the treating diagnosis (eg, a patient with a hip fracture also has chronic obstructive pulmonary disease); (2) complexities, a concomitant diagnosis related to the treating diagnosis (eg, a patient with rheumatoid arthritis undergoes a total shoulder replacement); or (3) complicating factors, issues that arise from the original diagnosis (eg, a postsurgical infection). Other issues that might impact the patient's participation with physical therapy and recovery that should be included are cognitive, psychological, social, and economic issues that might complicate or slow down the rehabilitative process. This information can be combined with the rehabilitation potential to provide a better picture of the therapist's expectations (Example 9-5).

Anticipated Goals and Expected Outcomes

The prognosis includes a list of goals or expected outcomes written to reflect the patient's final status at the end of the episode of care. They may be called outcome goals, expected outcomes, discharge goals, or long-term goals (LTGs). When writing a goal, the therapist determines the anticipated level of improvement based on the data and knowledge of the condition and the time required to reach this level. Perfecting goal-writing skills requires practice, and observing patient progression in a variety of circumstances helps in this process. Any component of the prognosis, including the outcome goals, may be modified at any point in the episode of care if the patient is progressing faster or slower than what was expected. A statement(s) that provides a justification for revising goals is included.

The Mechanics of Goal Writing

Well-written goals include 4 parts. As a guide, remember the ABCD of goal writing. "A" stands for *audience*, this is the individual who will be demonstrating the behavior or the attribute. In physical therapy, the "A" should be the patient or the patient's family member or caregiver. The "A" is *not* the therapist or another health care provider. "B" stands for *behavior*. The behavior is the action or attribute(s) being performed or assessed. A behavior might be a functional task such as walking, getting in or out of bed, or reaching. It might be learned information such as hip precautions. A behavior might also be a specific attribute the patient displays, such as muscle strength, blood pressure, or pain. "C" stands for *condition*. This includes a description of the conditions under which the behavior is to be performed. Conditions could include the environmental setting in which the behavior will be performed (eg, on level surfaces) or the presence or absence of assistive or adaptive equipment. "D" stands for *degree*. This is the degree to which the attribute should be demonstrated. This is a measurable term. A degree might be the specific muscle grade expected, the level of assist needed, the time it will take to complete a task, or the degree of accuracy expected.

The acronym SMART is also used to describe an appropriately structured goal. SMART stands for Specific, Measurable, Attainable, Realistic, and Timely. This acronym incorporates many of the components as outlined in the ABCD method, but it also highlights the concept of making sure the goals are attainable and realistic. This is important when the patient's prognosis is difficult to determine because of the complexity of the problems.

Whether the ABCD or SMART method is used, goals should always be specific and measurable to allow for ease in outcomes assessment, and they should paint a very clear picture of what the patient will look like at the end of the episode of care. As a rule of thumb, write a goal for every problem identified in the problem list (Example 9-6).

However, a single goal can be written to include multiple problems. When writing goals, one can address impairments, activity limitations, and/or participation restrictions. But, when writing a goal at the impairment level, relate it to a functional activity that will also be improved as the impairment is resolved (Example 9-7).

Integrating the Evidence Into Goal Writing

Several methods have been suggested to incorporate the evidence on an instrument's measurement properties into patient goals.[5,6] For example, a goal may reflect a value that would be considered "normal" for a particular test or measure. Goals may include relevant properties such as the instrument's minimal detectable change or the minimal clinically important difference. These values provide the amount of change that would be clinically relevant or clinically meaningful to the patient, respectively. Goals may include values that discriminate one population from another (eg, Berg Balance Score of 45 is indicative of fall risk)[7] or that coincide with a specific level of disability.[5] When specific values of an instrument are not known, the goal may be written so the degree of change exceeds the instrument's associated amount of error at minimum. One may also choose to examine prognostic studies for establishing an appropriate benchmark for a patient's goals. Using measurement properties in this manner requires the physical therapist be familiar with the current literature regarding the tests and measures used clinically that help to integrate evidence into practice.

MacDermid and Stratford[5] provided an example of a patient with rotator cuff disease. During an initial examination, a patient's score on the Disabilities of the Arm, Shoulder, and Hand Self-Report Questionnaire (DASH) was 44. In deciding goals for this patient, the physical therapist was also able to extrapolate from the literature that the minimal clinically important difference on the DASH was approximately 15 points. Therefore, he wrote the following outcome goal for the patient[5]:

In 12 weeks, the patient will demonstrate an important change in his DASH score (> 15 points).

The therapist knew from Beaton et al[8] that a score of 26.8 on the DASH coincided with a patient returning to work,[5] so the following goal was written:

In 3 months, the patient will demonstrate a DASH score < 25.

In this example, the therapist used the value reported in the literature that discriminates patients who are working vs those who are not. This could accompany a goal for the patient to return to work. Using the tool's measurement properties can help write goals and reflect meaningful clinical changes in a patient's status. In an ideal world, data on measurement tools would be easily available to clinicians; however, this is usually not the case, and clinicians may have to extrapolate from more general research

Example 9-6. Physical Therapy Assessment

A: 59-year-old man s/p fall at work sustaining a (R) rotator cuff tear 6 months ago; now 1 week following repair; physical therapy diagnosis is surgical restrictions as well as impaired ROM and strength limiting his ability to elevate arm overhead, reach overhead cabinets, perform normal home-management tasks, or perform work activities as a custodian. Pt. has type 2 diabetes that may slow progress but pt. reports motivation to return to work.

Physical Therapy Problems

*Impairments**

a.   Pain at rest and with activity
b.   Decreased ROM
c.   Decreased strength
d.   Healing surgical incision with ecchymosis

Activity Limitations and Participation Restrictions

a.   Moderate to severe difficulty on ADLs
b.   Unable to elevate arm overhead
c.   Severe difficulty sleeping due to pain

d.   Unable to manage transportation needs
e.   Unable to work
f.   Unable to participate in recreational activities
g.   DASH score 55/100

The pt. demonstrates good potential for full recovery and to meet physical therapy goals. In 16 weeks, the pt. will demonstrate:

a.   Pain < 3/10 to allow a full night's sleep[†]
b.   165° of shoulder flexion to allow full arm elevation to perform overhead activities[†]
c.   Strength in the shoulder girdle muscles 4/5 to allow full use upon RTW[†]
d.   Healed surgical scar with no complications
e.   Independent with and pain-free ADLs
f.   Independent in managing transportation needs
g.   Return to work with minimal to no limitations
h.   Full participation in recreational activities
i.   Final DASH score < 20

*The problem list can be broken down as shown here, or one list may be created.

[†]Note how this goal includes an impairment, but it is related to function. It also addresses at least 1 problem from the problem list.

---

findings.[5] Using measurement properties in documentation is discussed further in later chapters.

Establishing the Goal's Time Frame

The time it takes to reach the outcome goals is a clinical judgment made by the physical therapist. The time frame is set in terms of days, visits, weeks, or months. One important factor for consideration is the medical diagnosis. For example, the expectations for recovery are very different for a patient with a minor musculoskeletal condition vs one with a degenerative neuromuscular disorder. Other considerations include the particular setting, rehabilitation protocol, and time for tissue healing to occur. For example, a patient is recovering from a cerebrovascular accident and is receiving physical therapy services in an inpatient rehabilitation hospital. The physical therapist chooses to set the time frame on the outcome goals based on how long he suspects the patient will be in the unit (eg, 2 weeks). In another example, a patient undergoes an Achilles tendon repair; the physical therapist examines the patient, and, based on the established protocol and time for tissue healing, sets the time frame for 12 to 16 weeks. Example 9-8 provides examples of goals that are suitable for documentation in a patient's medical record.

Example 9-7. Addressing Function in Physical Therapy Goals

1. In 6 weeks, the pt. will demonstrate increased active hip extension to 20° **to allow normal prosthetic gait**.

2. In 3 months, the pt.'s strength will increase from 2/5 to 4/5 **to increase independence with sit-to-stand, transfers, and safe ambulation**.

3. In 6 visits, the pt.'s pain will decrease from 9/10 to 4/10 **to allow pt. to achieve a full night of sleep**.

Short-Term Goals

If there is a significant difference between the patient's current condition and the expected outcomes (outcome goals), the therapist may choose to include short-term goals (STGs). STGs serve as "bridge" goals between the patient's current status and the long-term expected outcome goals. Any STG written generally reflects a long-term, outcome goal. However, not all outcome goals have STGs and vice versa. STGs are desirable for several reasons. One reason is

Example 9-8. Including Timeframe in Physical Therapy Goals

1. In 3 days, the pt. will ambulate 50' with a standard walker 50% weight bearing on the (L) LE with close supervision on level surfaces.
2. In 6 weeks, the pt. will show increased shoulder flexion from 90° to 165° to allow improved overhead reaching.
3. In 3 weeks, the pt. will demonstrate normal vital signs after ambulating with supervision for 500'.
4. In 12 weeks, the pt.'s Berg Balance Test will increase to 50 indicating no longer at risk for falling.[7]
5. In 3 weeks, the pt.'s husband will be independent with assisting the pt. during car transfers.
6. In 6 weeks, the pt.'s quadriceps strength will increase from 3/5 to 4+/5 to allow improved ability to rise from the floor and stair climbing.
7. In 2 weeks, the child will be able to hold her head at midline while focusing on a toy for 1 minute.
8. In 3 days, the pt. will transfer from the bed to and from the wheelchair with minimal assist during sit-to-stand and to maintain weight-bearing precautions.
9. In 30 days, the pt. will be independent with home ambulation (~ 250') with a straight cane on carpet and hard surfaces.
10. The infant will bring both hands to midline without prompting in 6 weeks.
11. In 10 visits, the pt. will be able to have full finger ROM to allow full grip during home tasks and recreational activities.
12. In 4 weeks, the pt. will ambulate 500' on a variety of surfaces with a quad cane and supervision with a velocity exceeding 1.0 m/s.
13. In 6 weeks, the pt.'s Fugl-Meyer Upper Extremity score will improve 8% to 10%.[9]
14. In 4 weeks, the pt.'s score on the Foot and Ankle Ability measure will increase 9 to 10 points.[10]
15. In 6 weeks, the pt.'s score on the Penn Shoulder Scale will increase 15 points.[11]

Example 9-9. Short-Term Goals

1. The pt. will ambulate 50' with a standard walker 50% weight bearing on the (L) LE with close supervision on level surfaces.
   STG: The pt. will ambulate 25' with a standard walker non-weight bearing on the (L) LE with minimal assist of 1 for sequencing and balance in single-limb stance.
2. The pt. will show increased shoulder flexion from 90° to 165° to allow improved overhead reaching.
   STG: The pt. will show increased shoulder flexion from 90° to 120° to allow reaching into a low cabinet and improved ADL performance.
3. The pt. will demonstrate normal vital signs after ambulating with supervision for 500'.
   STG: The pt. will demonstrate normal vital signs after ambulating with contact guard assist of 1 for 100'.

to help guide the decision-making process. As the patient progresses through the episode of care, STGs are used as landmarks or stepping stones to help the therapist determine if the patient is making the desired/expected progress within a reasonable amount of time. Without STGs, it can be more difficult for the therapist to gauge if the patient is making satisfactory progress. STGs also provide an excellent recording mechanism for third-party payers to demonstrate the patient's response to the physical therapy plan of care. Third-party payers demand documentation that interventions are influencing the patient's problem(s), and STGs are a useful method to allow clear communication of the patient's progress. Finally, STGs provide a motivating factor for the patient. During a long-term rehabilitative process, patients can often become discouraged with what seems like little to no change from day to day, but STGs can provide small but realistic expectations and stepping stones on which the patient can focus. Example 9-9 provides examples of STGs.

> **Example 9-10. Amount, Frequency, and Duration**
>
> Discharge Goals:
> 1. The pt. will demonstrate decreased pain from 7/10 to 2/10 in 4 weeks to allow pain-free ambulation.
> 2. The pt. will be independent in all transfers in 8 weeks.
> 3. The pt. will return home to live independently in 8 weeks.
>
> Plan: The pt. will be seen twice daily, 6 days per week, for the next 8 weeks.

> **Example 9-11. Plans for Skills Care**
>
> 1. Skilled services will be provided to educate the pt. on surgical precautions, assist in performing safe transfers, instruct and assist in weight-bearing precautions and use of assistive device, and provide a safe exercise progression to improve motion and strength.
> 2. Skilled services will be provided to design and implement safe activities to promote normal trunk and head alignment, to instruct the parents in proper handling skills to decrease tone, and to educate parents on adaptive seating.

THE INTERVENTION PLAN

The Amount, Frequency, and Duration

The overall plan of care will include a clear statement of the intervention plan. In the SOAP note format, this information is documented in the Plan (P:) section of the note. Documentation of the intervention plan includes the amount, frequency, and duration of services the patient will need to achieve the established goals and outcomes. In an inpatient setting, this might be twice daily for the next 3 to 4 days or 1 time daily, 5 times per week, for the next 4 weeks. In skilled nursing settings, it is important that the amount and frequency, or total therapy minutes, correspond with the patient's corresponding "RUG level." This will be discussed more in later chapters. In an outpatient setting, this may read 3 times per week for 6 weeks or twice weekly for 3 months. Although some goals will be met sooner than others, in general, it is important that the duration of services provided in the plan matches the longest time frame written on the discharge goals (Example 9-10).

The duration of services in Example 9-10 matches the time frame set on goal 3, which is the time in which the physical therapist thinks the patient will be discharged from the facility. Note the time frame on goal 1 is for 4 weeks. It is assumed once this is achieved, the therapist will be working toward the other established goals.

Plan for Skilled Care

It is important when documenting the plan of care to include a statement summarizing the plan for skilled services. This is a statement(s) that provides an overview of the therapist's skills the patient needs to achieve the desired outcomes. It serves as a general statement to indicate the skilled care to be provided and "sets the stage" for the more specific list of interventions that will follow. It is important to use the term *skilled services* in this section. Skills indicated in this aspect of the note can include education, safety, progression, etc. This is an area of documentation that is still emerging and often difficult to articulate. In using the SOAP structure, one may find this statement in the A: aspect of the note. Example 9-11 shows how this important piece of information can be provided.

Specific Services to Be Provided

The plan also includes a detailed list of specific interventions that will be provided. This list includes the scientific rationale for providing the specific intervention(s) to show medical necessity. Interventions include any purposeful interaction that will occur between the physical therapist or physical therapist assistant and the patient or caregiver that is designed to facilitate change (and meet the stated goals). Examples include patient education, therapeutic exercise, and functional training. As noted in Chapter 4, the *Guide to Physical Therapist Practice*[3] lists 9 categories of interventions. Each category further includes several specific types of interventions (eg, specific types of therapeutic exercises include gait and locomotor training, stretching exercises, and relaxation techniques, to name just a few). When documenting the interventions, it is important to include enough detail to describe *what* will be done and *why* it will be done; however, the therapist should avoid writing the plan in a way that will require unnecessary frequent updates or modifications. For example, the physical therapist might indicate electrotherapeutic agents will be used to address pain, but specific parameters should not be included. This will allow the therapist to choose between different devices and alter the parameters without the necessity of updating the plan of care each time. This will also allow the physical therapist assistant to make appropriate modifications for patient progression and comfort without the necessity of consulting with the physical therapist regarding every slight modification.

Example 9-12. Specific Planned Interventions and Rationale

Specific Interventions:

1. Hip and knee therapeutic exercise to improve ROM and strength to improve ambulation and transfers.
2. Gait training to improve home mobility, safety, and (I) living.
3. Transfer training to promote home independence and safety with weight-bearing restrictions.
4. Discuss home equipment needs with case manager.

In addition to planned interventions, the plan of care should include any planned collaboration with other health care providers necessary to meet the patient's goals. For example, if during the examination process the physical therapist determines the patient's medication regimen is impacting the patient's responses negatively, he or she will document a plan to discuss these issues with the physician.

The importance of patient education within the intervention cannot be overstated. It is through the educational process that the patient and the patient's family or caregiver are assisted in taking full and complete ownership of the patient's health and well-being. Helping patients develop the knowledge, skills, and attitudinal framework necessary to manage their own health care concerns moves them to independence. Patient-related instruction can encompass several different topics, including education about (1) the pathology/disease process, (2) the body structure or body function impairments, (3) functional limitations, (4) how those impairments and functional limitations impact the patient's participation within social roles, (5) the physical therapy plan of care, (6) general health issues such as the patient's need for a fitness program or information regarding appropriate nutrition, (7) a home exercise program, (8) home or work modifications, (9) functional task training, (10) precautions or restrictions, and (11) appropriate activity level based on the pathology.[3] Within the plan, document specific topics and information that will be provided to a patient. For example, a patient who is recovering from a total hip arthroplasty will require targeted information related to hip arthroplasty precautions. Goals may be written that reflect specific aspects of patient education and that patient learning has occurred (Example 9-12).

In some instances, the plan may also state the date of the next formal reassessment or re-evaluation and give the discharge plan(s). Discharge plans may include transfer to another setting for further physical therapy services (eg, transfer from acute care hospital to a skilled nursing facility) or discharge to a home maintenance program (Example 9-13).

HOW A PHYSICAL THERAPIST ASSISTANT USES THE ASSESSMENT AND PLAN (PLAN OF CARE)

The diagnosis, prognosis, and intervention plan, documented within the plan of care (Assessment and Plan sections of the SOAP note), are of vital importance for the physical therapist assistant. The assistant reviews the assessment to find out the reason for therapy services, the specific problems to be addressed, issues that may influence the intervention, and the anticipated goals. The assistant reviews the plan to identify the interventions that will be provided. The Plan section is of particular importance because it provides the guideline(s) for the interventions the assistant can legally perform. For example, a physical therapist directs the assistant to work with a patient on functional mobility. The assistant reviews the Assessment section to understand the patient's diagnosis, mobility problems, and prognosis. This will help the assistant have appropriate and realistic expectations and be able to anticipate the patient's responses to the interventions. The physical therapist assistant references the plan to determine specific mobility skills to address and parameters in which he or she can legally progress the patient because the assistant can adjust the interventions only within the guidelines documented within the plan. The assistant also references the plan when he or she feels a patient's interventions should be adjusted (Example 9-14).

In Example 9-14, the physical therapist has identified the assistive device, interventions, and functional training this patient will receive. If this were a real plan, then a physical therapist assistant could *not* advance the assistive device to a cane, and the physical therapist assistant could *not* perform strengthening exercises because these are not part of the established plan. However, an assistant could choose the range of motion exercises and the mobility training because these are less prescriptive. The amount of detail provided in a plan determines how the physical therapist assistant can progress the patient. If the patient's response to interventions is not as anticipated (whether the patient is not responding to the established plan or if the patient's progression is more rapid than expected), the physical therapist assistant can inform the physical therapist and request alterations to the plan of care.

When reviewing the Assessment and Plan sections of the SOAP note, the assistant will have the following questions in mind[12]:

- What interventions does the physical therapist want me to provide?
- What problem(s) is the intervention addressing?

Example 9-13. Plan 1

P: The pt. will be seen 2 times per week for the next 12 to 6 weeks. Skilled care will be provided to educate pt. on precautions, safe progression of therapeutic exercises, appropriate use of sling and abduction pillow, and to educate spouse on assistance during home exercises. For the next 5 weeks, the pt. will receive (1) passive ROM to improve flexion, abduction, IR, and ER to allow full capsular mobility and prevent adhesive capsulitis since the pt. is at risk because of diabetes; (2) modalities to control pain; (3) active scapular exercises to promote scapulothoracic mobility; and (4) instruction in a home exercise program. In 6 weeks, there will be a reassessment to determine the appropriate interventions at that time that will allow him to meet the above goals and return to his prior status including RTW.

Example 9-14. Plan 2

P: Skilled services will be provided to educate the pt. on use of a standard walker, to provide cueing during ambulation for safety and weight-bearing precautions, and to perform ROM exercises to improve knee and hip mobility allowing the pt. to ascend and descend stairs and sit comfortably. The pt. will also receive functional mobility training to improve safety and independence so that she can return to living independently at home. Pt. will be seen 2 times per day for 3 to 5 days.

- What is the patient's current status regarding this condition?
- What are the physical therapist's and patient's goals?
- What is the patient's diagnosis?
- What is the patient's prognosis?
- Are there any contraindications or precautions I need to keep in mind?
- Are there any other special issues I need to keep in mind?

THE ASSESSMENT AND PLAN IN AN ELECTRONIC MEDICAL RECORD

Templates of a physical therapy electronic medical record often consist of a series of drop-down menus and checkboxes to facilitate ease of documentation. There are often templates for many aspects of the Assessment and Plan sections, or plan of care. There may be a list of choices for establishing the problem list: checkboxes for rehabilitation potential, checkboxes for factors that influence treatment, a list of pre-established goals, checkboxes for the interventions to be provided, and checkboxes for the amount, frequency, and duration of services. When documenting using predetermined lists or choices in this manner, it is easy to rapidly overselect or get into a habit of selecting the same choices for all patients. This, along with the "canned" phrases generated by some software programs, can quickly limit the individual nature of the problem list and often does not reflect a patient's unique problems, functional demands, and lifestyle. In addition, it is difficult to articulate the need for skilled care and

medical necessity of the interventions using predetermined checkboxes and lists. With the ubiquitous nature of the use of the electronic medical record, one must be cognizant of these issues and create documentation that includes the necessary components of contemporary documentation, captures a patient's unique status and needs, and maintains patient individuality within the diagnosis, problems list, goals, and interventions.

SUMMARY

At the onset of physical therapy services, it is imperative that documentation outlines the findings from the examination and evaluation and includes a detailed plan of care. The SOAP note is a common documentation format that can be used for this process. The SOAP format outlines the findings from the examination in the Subjective and Objective sections and details the evaluation, diagnosis, prognosis, and interventions within the Assessment and Plan sections (Figure 9-3). This initial documentation provides the format and foundational information on which all future physical therapy sessions are based. All future documentation should refer to the structure and information provided within the initial note (see Figure 9-2; see also Figures 4-1, 5-3, and 5-4).

REVIEW QUESTIONS

1. List the information found within the Assessment and Plan sections of the SOAP note.
2. Describe the relationship between the examination and the evaluation.
3. Differentiate between a linear clinical decision-making model and a dynamic clinical decision-making model. Which model best describes the process often used within the physical therapy evaluative process?
4. How should the physical therapist construct a physical therapy diagnosis?

Figure 9-3. Relationship between the Patient/Client Management Model and the SOAP note format.

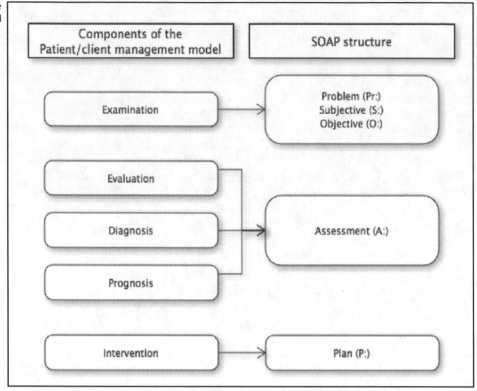

5. List some considerations for developing a prognosis.

6. List and describe the components of a well-written goal.

7. How can a physical therapist integrate evidence regarding tests and measures into goal statements?

8. How does the physical therapist assistant use the information documented in the Assessment and Plan sections of a SOAP note? How can the therapist structure the note to enhance the physical therapist/physical therapist assistant relationship?

9. Outline an appropriate structure for the documentation of the Assessment and Plan sections of a SOAP note.

APPLICATION EXERCISES

1. Read the following goals and identify the audience, behavior, condition, and degree. Also, identify missing components. When appropriate, determine if the goal addresses an impairment (I), an activity limitation (AL), or a participation restriction (PR).

a. STG: Decreased turgor and fibrosis by 50% (to a 7×15 cm area) within 4 to 6 visits.

b. STG: Decrease girth of (R) ankle to within 1 cm of (L) (using figure 8) in 3 visits.

c. LTG: The patient will demonstrate mastery of pacing and other overuse reduction strategies to allow him to return to work.

d. STG: Decrease pain to 3/10 during movement.

e. LTG: Patient will display normal gait pattern.

f. LTG: In 4 to 6 weeks, the patient will be (I) with bed mobility & transfers including supine to and from sit, w/c to and from bed (no sliding board), and w/c to and from floor.

g. LTG: In 4 to 6 weeks, the patient will be (I) with w/c mobility on level surfaces, up and down curbs, and on uneven surfaces.

h. STG: The patient will verbalize 3/3 hip precautions without verbal prompts.

i. LTG: In 8 weeks, the patient will participate in a community outing with only min (A) of 1.

j. STG: The wound will have an area of 2×2 cm with 1-cm depth.

2. Match the appropriate short-term goal for the following outcome goals.

Outcome goal	Short-term goals (STGs)
_____1. The patient will ambulate with prosthesis 500' without assistive device on varied terrain with close supervision in 6 weeks.	A. The patient will manage his wheelchair on a variety of surfaces 250' with minimal verbal cueing in 2 weeks.
_____2. The patient will transfer to and from all surfaces with supervision in 2 weeks.	B. The patient will transfer to and from the right independently and to and from the left with minimal assist of 1 in 3 to 5 days.
_____3. The patient will manage his wheelchair independently for 500' in an open environment to allow independent community mobility in 1 month.	C. The patient will ambulate 75' with a standard walker and the prosthesis with minimal assist of 1 for balance and weight shifting in 3 weeks.
_____4. The patient will ambulate 150' with prosthesis and standard walker on level surface independently in 6 weeks.	D. The patient will propel his wheelchair on level surfaced 50-75' with verbal cues in 2 weeks.
_____5. The patient will manage his wheelchair 100' on level surfaces and small inclines independently in 4 weeks.	E. The patient will ambulate 250' with prosthesis and quad cane on level surfaces and small inclines with supervision and verbal cues in 3 weeks.

3. Given the following data provided in an initial examination, write a goal if the expectation is that the patient will improve.

Strength: 5/5 throughout (B) LEs except (R) quadriceps 3/5 because of pain and (R) hamstrings 3/5 because of disuse.

AROM	Left	Right
DF	0 to 20 degrees	−5 degrees from neutral
PF	0 to 40 degrees	5 degrees

Mobility: Bed mobility: rolling with mod (A) ×1 and frequent verbal cues for sequencing and setup.

Transfers: Bed/mat to and from w/c with max (A) of 1 to 2, dependent with all setup.

Example 9-15. Assessment and Plan From Initial Documentation

Assessment:
59-year-old woman 2 weeks s/p fall injuring right knee and development of pneumonia; hospitalized x 5 days
Problem List
1. Knee pain
2. Limited ROM
3. Limited strength
4. Gait disturbance
STGs: 2 weeks
1. Decrease pain
2. Increase strength by one full grade
3. Increase AROM, PROM, and hamstring length by 20° and gastroc 10°
4. WNL gait pattern
LTGs: Resume maximum function of the (L) knee and discharge to home
Plan: PT bid for ROM and gait until discharge. Add strengthening exercises when pain decreases.

Gait: Patient ambulated 50' with small-based quad cane and mod (A) ×1 to assist with upright posture and increasing step length. Patient displayed ataxia, motor planning, and motor sequencing deficits.

4. Review the Assessment and Plan sections of the note as found in Example 9-15. Critique the note using the following questions.

    a. Does the note provide a physical therapy diagnosis?

    b. Does the note clearly demonstrate the clinical decision-making process?

    c. Does the note draw correlations between information about impairment and function?

    d. Does the note demonstrate the relationship between the problem list, the goals, and the interventions?

    e. Are the interventions clearly detailed to guide the physical therapist assistant?

5. Example 9-16 is the initial Subjective and Objective documentation for a patient recently admitted to an acute care hospital. Use it to complete the Assessment and Plan sections of the note.

Example 9-16. Subjective and Objective Sections of SOAP Note

Initial Evaluation

Date: 08/10/18

Pr: (L) CVA, (R) hemiplegia; HPI: 67-year-old male was admitted to acute care 08/08/18 because of sudden weakness in his (R) UE & LE and slurred speech. PMH: NIDDM, HTN, CABG ×2 07/05/2011. Height: 6'2", Weight 255 lbs, no other pertinent medical history. Current medications include Glucophage and captopril.

S: C/C: Inability to move, function, care for himself; weakness in (R) UE & LE; pain in the (R) shoulder 5/10. Prior Level of Function: (I) with all ADLs, IADLs, and gait without assistive device. Active; worked in his workshop, yard, and garden; performed all necessary home management tasks. His is (R) hand dominant. Home Situation: Retired carpenter; lives with his wife who is healthy but is a small woman. Live in 2-level home with 4 steps to enter. Pt.'s Goals: Return to prior lifestyle.

O: Systems Review: CP System: HR, 96 bpm; BP, 128/88; RR, 14. Integumentary System: (+) edema, no other abnormalities noted. Neuromuscular and Musculoskeletal Systems: Impairments identified, see Tests and Measures below. Cognition/Communication: Slurred speech. Alter and oriented x 4.

Tests/Measures: Observations: 3+ pitting edema (R) hand and forearm; tendency to keep (R) in dependent position. Figure 8 Hand Girth: (R) 54 cm, (L) 52 cam. Capillary Refill: Normal. Sensation: Diminished light touch, deep pressure localization, proprioception & kinesthesia through the (R) UE & LE. Muscle Tone: Diminished tone on (R) UE & LE to passive range. Reflexes: diminished patellar reflex and absent Achilles reflex on (R). Shoulder: 1 finger width sulcus at (R) GH joint. Balance: Unable to stand without physical assistance or UE support. Endurance: Tolerated 30-minute session requiring 1-minute rest break every 5 to 8 minutes. Functional Status: Bed Mobility: Max (A) x 1 scooting up/down and side/side in bed; mod (A) rolling supine to/from sit min (A) x 1 from (R) and mod (A) from (L); sit to/from stand mod (A) x 2; stand pivot w/c to/from bed mod (A) x 2. Posture: Trunk in laterally flexed position and slightly rotated to the left. Gait: Ambulated in // x 8' x 2 with mod (A) x 2. Required 2 to stabilize and balance at the trunk and 1 for assisting with advancing the (R) LE and stabilizing the (R) UE; required verbal cues for sequencing as pt. very impulsive during gait. W/C Management: Dependent in parts and mobility. Strength:

	RIGHT	LEFT
Shoulder		
Flexion	2—/5	5/5
Extension	2—/5	5/5
Abduction	2—/5	5/5
IR/ER	2—/5	5/5
Elbow		
Flexion	2—/5	5/5
Extension	2—/5	5/5
Wrist		
Flexion	2—/5	5/5
Extension	2—/5	5/5
Finger		
Flexion	1/5	5/5
Hip		
Flexion	3—/5	5/5
Extension	3—/5	5/5
Abduction	3+/5	5/5
Adduction	3+/5	5/5
IR/ER	3+/5	5/5
Knee		
Flexion	3+/5	5/5
Extension	3—/5	5/5
Ankle		
DF	2—/5	5/5
PF	2—/5	5/5

REFERENCES

1. Jones M. Clinical reasoning in manual therapy. *Phys Ther.* 1992;72:43-52.
2. Centers for Medicare & Medicaid Services. Covered medical and other health services. *Medicare Benefit Policy Manual.* Publication 1 00-02. https://www.cms.gov/Regulations-and-Guidance/Guidance/Manuals/Downloads/bp102c15.pdf. Accessed May 3, 2019
3. American Physical Therapy Association. *Guide to Physical Therapist Practice.* 2016. http://guidetoptpractice.apta.org/. Accessed April 18, 2018.
4. Cunningham C, Horgan F, O'Neill D. Clinical assessment of rehabilitation potential of the older patient: a pilot study. *Clin Rehabil.* 2000;14:205-207.
5. MacDermid J, Stratford P. Applying evidence on outome mesaures to hand therapy practice. *J Hand Ther.* 2004;17:165-173.
6. Martin R, Irrgang J, Burdett R, Conti S, Van Swearingen J. Evidence of validity for the Foot and Ankle Ability Measure. *Foot Ankle Int.* 2006;26:968-983.
7. Riddle D, Stratford P. Intepreting validity indexes for diagnostic tests: an illustration using the Berg Balance Test. *Phys Ther.* 1999;79:939-948.
8. Beaton D, Datz J, Fossel A, Wright J, Tarasuk V. Measuring the whole or parts: validity, reliability, and responsivness of the DASH outcome measure in different regions of the upper extremity. *J Hand Ther.* 2001;14:128-146.
9. Page S, Fulk G, Boyne P. Clinically imprtant differences for the Upper-Extremity Fugl Meyer Scale in people with minimal to moderate impairment due to chronic stroke. *Phys Ther.* 2012;92:791-798.
10. Martin R, Irrgang J. A survey of self-reported outcome instruments for the foot and ankle. *J Orthop Sports Phys Ther.* 2007;37:72-84.
11. Leggin B, Michener L, Shaffer M, Brenneman S, Iannotti J, Williams G. The Penn Shoulder Score: reliability and validity. *J Orthop Sports Phys Ther.* 2006;36:138-151.
12. Erickson ML, McKnight R. *Documentation Basics for the Physical Therapist Assistant.* 3rd ed. Thorofare, NJ: SLACK Incorporated; 2018.

APPENDIX 9-1: TIPS FOR DOCUMENTING SPECIFIC INFORMATION

Tips for documenting results of tests and measures:

- When documenting results of data collection, include all information needed for the test to be reproduced and for the results to be clearly understood. Be sure to include the following:
  - Procedure used (eg, goniometry, MMT, and observation)
  - Exactly what was measured (eg, right elbow flexion PROM)
  - The patient's position

Types of information related to tests and measures:

A variety of test procedures and observations are used when measuring the patient's status and response to interventions. Test are performed at both the body structure and function level (eg, ROM and MMT) as well as the activity and participation level (eg, bed mobility and gait). The following is a list of common tests and observations and delineates components that should be documented for each:

1. Vital signs (indicate before and/or after exercise/activity as appropriate)
   - Heart rate
     - Location
     - Quality
     - Rate
   - Respiratory rate
     - Rate
     - Rhythm
     - Depth
     - Regularity of pattern
   - Blood pressure
     - Location, side
     - Systolic over diastolic (eg, BP: [R] brachial 120/80)
2. Anthropometric characteristics
   - Height
   - Weight
   - Length
   - Girth
3. Muscle strength
   - The measurement range (eg, when documenting strength for right elbow flexors, document 3/5 instead of 3)
   - What is measured
     - Muscle group (eg, hip flexors)
     - Specific muscles (eg, gluteus maximus)
     - Arrange logically (group per anatomical location; eg, group shoulder musculature together: shoulder flexors 4/5, extensors 4–/5, abduction 4–/5, adduction 4+/5)
     - Use tables or columns to show (B) measurement or before/after measurements
   - Any deviation from standard position/protocol (eg, tested hip extension in side-lying due to the patient being unable to tolerate the prone position because of obesity)
4. Pain
   - Results from written pain questionnaires, scales, and diagrams (eg, McGill Pain Questionnaire, Pain Disability Index, visual analogue scales, pain drawings, and pain maps)
   - Note: verbal descriptions of pain given by the patient are often included in the subjective portion of the note. Sometimes data from pain questionnaires are also recorded in the subjective portion of the interim note.

- Describe patient's nonverbal pain responses to activities, positioning, and postures

5. Range of motion
   - Document the range from the beginning of the range available to the end of the range available (eg, elbow flexion 5 to 110 degrees instead of just elbow flexion 110 degrees)
   - Specific joint
   - Arrange logically
   - Group per anatomical location
   - Use tables or columns to show (B) measurements or before/after measurements
   - Any deviation from standard position/protocol (eg, shoulder external rotation; unable to achieve standard test position due to pain restrictions; pt. placed in 45 degrees of abduction for measurement)

6. Results of any standard tests or questionnaires
   - Record measurements per the standard of the test being used (eg, Berg Balance Test)

7. Assistive, adaptive, orthotic, protective, supportive, and prosthetic devices
   - Specify device being used (eg, left custom ankle-foot orthosis [AFO])
   - Discuss patient's (patient's family's/caregiver's) ability to care for device
   - Discuss patient's ability to don/doff device as appropriate
   - Discuss skin condition related to use of the device
   - Discuss safety risks associated with use of the device

8. Gait, locomotion, and balance
   - Indicate activity (eg, gait or wheelchair mobility)
   - Indicate any assistive, adaptive, orthotic, protective, supportive, or prosthetic devices used; for example, wheeled walker
   - Indicate type of surface the patient is traversing (eg, level surface or stairs)
   - Indicate distance traveled or amount of time activity is tolerated (eg, 100 feet or 10 minutes)
   - List amount and type of physical assistance provided (eg, patient required minimal assistance to place left lower extremity)
   - Number of people needed to aid (eg, patient required minimal assistance of 2 people); if no number is provided, then assume it is one person
   - List amount and type of cues given; for example, patient required constant verbal cues for cane placement
   - Describe gait pattern used if appropriate (eg, 4-point gait pattern)
   - Describe gait deviations if appropriate (eg, patient demonstrated left foot drop during swing phase of gait)
   - When documenting gait include weight-bearing status

9. Self-care, home management, and community or work reintegration
   - Record measurements of physical environments
   - Record any safety concerns or barriers in home, community, and work environments

10. Results of any standard tests or questionnaires
    - Record measurements per the standard of the test being used (eg, Functional Independence Measure [FIM] and SF-36)

Adapted from Erickson ML, McKnight R. *Documentation Basics for the Physical Therapist Assistant.* 3rd ed. Thorofare, NJ: SLACK Incorporated; 2018.

CHAPTER 10

Interim Documentation

Rebecca S. McKnight, PT, MS and Mia L. Erickson, PT, EdD

CHAPTER OUTLINE

- Treatment and Progress Notes
  - Subjective
  - Objective
  - Assessment
  - Assessing Change
  - Plan
  - Timing Interim Notes
- Re-evaluations
- Letters

CHAPTER OBJECTIVES

Upon completion of this chapter, the reader will be able to:
1. Describe the types of documentation that occur across the episode of care
2. List the various types of interim documentation
3. Discuss the roles of the physical therapist and the physical therapist assistant in documenting interim notes
4. Differentiate between a treatment note and a progress note
5. Document the intervention aspect of an interim note
6. Identify factors that would indicate the need for a re-evaluation
7. Discuss the relationship between the initial documentation and interim notes
8. Describe the contents of a letter to a physician
9. Integrate evidence in clinical decision making when examining patient change
10. Construct a progress note

Erickson ML, Utzman RR, McKnight RS.
Physical Therapy Documentation: From Examination to Outcome,
Third Edition (pp 97-107).
© 2020 Taylor & Francis Group.

KEY TERMS

episode of care
interim note
progress note (report)
reassessment
re-evaluation
treatment note

KEY ABBREVIATIONS

MCID
MDC
SEM

Physical therapy documentation occurs over the patient's entire episode of care. The physical therapy record clearly describes (1) the patient's condition, or pathology; (2) impairments in body structures and body functions; (3) functional or activity limitations and participation restrictions; (4) the physical therapist's clinical reasoning and rationale; (5) anticipated goals and expected outcomes; (6) skilled interventions provided, including patient education, communication with other disciplines, and specific procedural interventions; and (7) the final outcome, or result of the intervention.

The American Physical Therapy Association's Guidelines for Physical Therapy Documentation of Patient/Client Management indicates that documentation is required for every patient visit/encounter.[1] The documentation begins at the time of the initial visit with the examination and evaluation and continues during each visit/encounter through interim notes. Documentation concludes with the discharge summary, or note, following the last encounter in the episode of care (see Chapter 11). Notes written between the initial documentation and discharge note are called interim notes. Interim notes are written in the form of treatment or daily notes, progress notes, regular or formal reassessments, or re-evaluations. In order to demonstrate continuity of care being provided and to demonstrate the clinical decision-making process, each interim note refers to and is consistent with the initial documentation and any prior reassessments or re-evaluations. Interim notes help tell the patient's "story," and a reader should be able to follow the patient's progress while reading the record. It is also important that each interim note include enough detail to support the skilled interventions provided that day and provide justification for any new, medically necessary interventions added.

TREATMENT AND PROGRESS NOTES

The primary purposes of a treatment or daily note are to document what occurred during a session or encounter in relation to the skilled services provided and to support the billing codes that were used for that particular day. However, progress notes are more extensive and provide more data and detail in all sections, especially the Assessment and Plan. Progress notes provide changes to the plan of care, address the patient's goals, highlight patient progress, justify the need for continuing skilled care, and show care is reasonable and necessary. Any information typically required for a progress note may be included in a regular treatment note at any point in the episode of care, but it is not necessary. However, including more detail in treatment notes does help show improvement between the initial documentation and written progress notes. Recall from Chapter 4 that the Centers for Medicare & Medicaid Services has specific guidelines for treatment notes when treating Medicare beneficiaries in an outpatient setting. Anyone providing services to these individuals should review these guidelines on a regular basis because they do change. Also, anyone providing care to Medicare beneficiaries in other settings should be familiar with the documentation requirements for that setting. For learning note writing, the following rules can be used and then adapted by setting if needed.

Subjective

When writing, the Subjective section of interim notes (treatment of progress notes) includes patient (family member or caregiver) comments that are consistent with and address the chief complaints or issues noted in the initial documentation. Also, include patient daily comments and remarks regarding progress, effects of the intervention, functional changes, and status toward his or her goals. Show disablement concepts by detailing how the intervention has brought about changes in patient function, activity limitations, and participation restrictions using the patient's words. Provide, from the patient's perspective, how resolution of impairments is leading to improved function. Finally, include any new complaints, problems, or information relevant to the patient's current condition. Look at the following examples found in the Subjective section of a treatment or progress note:

1. Comments regarding patient status
   a. Patient reported working with his employer regarding return to work. Feeling like he can return to modified duty soon.
   b. Patient's wife stated she feels they can manage at home with some assistance from their children.
   c. Patient reported, "I am feeling stronger."
   d. Patient reported she was able to put the dishes into the cabinet last night for the first time since surgery.

e. The patient has been a widow for several years and lived alone prior to the accident; however, today reported her husband is waiting in her room to take her dancing.

f. Patient reported she can ambulate more independently in her home and her fear of falling is decreasing.

g. The patient's mother reported the patient continues to have problems with wheelchair mobility.

2. Patient's reaction to interventions provided

a. Patient states her pain level increased after her last therapy session when a new stretching activity was initiated, but she reports the increase in pain lasted only about one hour and then the pain returned to its normal level.

b. Patient reports relief of pain symptoms from 7/10 to 3/10 with the transcutaneous electrical nerve stimulation trial following the last visit that allowed her to achieve a full night of sleep.

c. The patient reported use of the straight cane has allowed her to be steadier during gait.

d. Patient's mother reports the patient is using the involved hand to reach for objects with less cueing.

e. Patient stated gait and balance training have helped. States she can now ambulate without assistance 1000', allowing her to ambulate from the car into her church service independently.

f. Patient's husband indicated the leg strengthening exercises have helped in that the patient is now able to transfer in and out of bed without assistance.

3. New problem(s) or new complaint(s)

a. Patient indicated that over the weekend he noticed increased redness and pain in the lower posterior calf and was diagnosed with a blood clot. States he has not been able to participate in therapy for the last 2 days.

b. Patient's mother reported a red spot on the right wrist after wearing the orthosis for 2 hours.

c. Patient complains of increased swelling after the addition of the strengthening exercises last session.

d. Patient complains of hip pain after initiating the ankle-foot orthosis last visit.

e. The nurse reported the patient developed a fever last night, and she thinks the incision may be infected.

f. The patient's wife reported an increase in difficulty breathing and wheezing following the increased activity in the last session.

4. Pertinent information not previously documented

a. A physical therapist in an outpatient setting has been working with a 48-year-old man who injured his back while moving. On the third visit, he informs the therapist he had a hernia repair 2 years ago. This information was not included in the initial evaluation or any of the subsequent interim notes.

Document: Patient indicated today that he had a hernia repair 2 years ago.

b. A physical therapist has been working with an 8-year-old boy in the school system. He has spastic diplegia, and a goal is to ambulate between the classroom and cafeteria with supervision and a posterior walker. Today the student tells the therapist that he has started walking with his parents in the evening on a high school track. Document: Today patient reported he has been walking with his parents on a local track.

In most cases, do not use subheadings when writing the Subjective section of interim notes (treatment or progress) but, rather, organize the section by logically grouping together similar information. For example, all information related to the patient's pain (rating, description, and behavior) is grouped together, and information related to home environment (distance needed to walk, steps to negotiate, and type of flooring) is grouped together. However, it is advisable to use subheadings to organize information when there are many pieces of subjective data such as in a progress note. Anytime subheadings are included, use those that are consistent with the initial documentation. This will assist the reader in following patient comments throughout the episode of care.

Objective

When writing, the Objective section of interim notes includes (1) results of any screenings, tests, measures, and observations; (2) the patient's functional status; and (3) a clear description of the interventions that are consistent with what is billed on that day of service. In a progress note, the Objective section includes more data and is more thorough than a typical treatment note. When documenting the objective, show consistency by using measures that are consistent with those on the initial and prior documentation. Provide results of any new screenings, tests, and measures when appropriate to show progress (or lack of) toward the established goals.

Document the patient's functional status, including the function, distance or time, type and amount of skilled assistance required, type and amount of cues provided, quality of movement, weight-bearing status, condition under which the function is performed (eg, surfaces), barriers, safety concerns, and any other relevant information to create a clear picture. It is imperative to include the type of assistance provided, especially when a unique or complex skill is used to assist the patient. This helps in showing that skilled assistance was provided. Record functional status, especially in areas for which there is an established goal. This allows the reader to see progress made toward goals and that these areas are being addressed during the treatment sessions.

To document interventions, record any information that would allow another therapist to replicate the session. Specific information often includes the following:

- The intervention, which falls into one of the following categories[2]:
  - Patient or client instruction (used with every patient and client)
  - Airway clearance techniques (eg, forced expiratory techniques, assisted coughing, drainage, and breathing techniques)
  - Assistive technology (aids for locomotion, orthoses, prosthesis, seating and positioning devices, and transfer aids)
  - Biophysical agents (eg, electrical stimulation, biofeedback, iontophoresis, ultrasound, heat, ice, whirlpool, laser, ultraviolet, compression, and standing frames)
  - Functional training in self-care and domestic, work, community, social, and civic life (eg, self-care, home management, work, community, school, play, recreation)
  - Integumentary repair and protective techniques (eg, wound care, scar management, debridement of necrotic tissue, and dressings)
  - Manual therapy techniques (eg, lymphatic draining, manual traction, massage, soft tissue or joint mobilization, and passive stretching)
  - Motor function training
  - Therapeutic exercise (eg, aerobic or endurance training, balance training, postural training, developmental activities, range of motion, flexibility, motor training, and strengthening)
- Side and body part (eg, spine, right shoulder, and left knee)
- Patient position (eg, prone or side lying) when not performed in the standard position
- Dosage (eg, frequency, intensity, duration, sets, repetitions, settings, and parameters)
- Equipment used (eg, weights, assistive or adaptive devices, spirometer, and traction device)
- Rest breaks
- A rationale for the intervention if being performed for the first time
- Time for each intervention
- Total treatment time

Use subheadings to clearly differentiate between tests and measures, the patient's functional status, and the interventions provided. When using electronic documentation or standard forms, these sections are divided automatically; however, when writing interim notes by hand or free typing, clearly differentiate these important aspects of the Objective section.

Document any communication or collaboration with other health care providers or agencies involved in the patient's care, such as personal, phone, or electronic conversations, team meetings, case management, and discharge planning. Document education (patient, family, caregiver, etc) intended to optimize the intervention.[2] Education often relates to the pathology, impairments, activity limitations, participation restrictions, the plan of care, transition to a different role or setting, risk factors, health or wellness needs, precautions, restrictions, safety, and home exercises.[2] Document the specific education that occurred, the type (verbal, handout, brochure, etc), and the patient's (family member's/caregiver's) response to the education. Maintain copies of all written materials provided to patients. Additionally, document the presence of learning barriers.

Assessment

Use the Assessment section of the interim Subjective, Objective, Assessment, and Plan (SOAP) note to summarize the relevance of data documented within the Subjective and Objective sections. Highlight, or summarize, changes in the patient's status for that day of service (ie, pre- and posttreatment) or since the last visit, the initial session, or the last reassessment. These changes include improvements made in impairments, activity limitations, or participation restrictions. When applicable, describe how the physical therapy interventions have helped in bringing about these changes. In the event the patient's status has not changed (ie, plateaued) or has shown a decline in status, use the assessment to describe this plateau or decline and provide a rationale. Like with other sections of the SOAP note, the Assessment section of the progress note is much more extensive and addresses all patient change (or lack thereof) up to that point in the episode of care or since the last progress note. The amount of patient change summarized in a treatment note is an individual therapist decision. For example, a physical therapist may choose to focus on highlighting change in 1 or 2 patient problems in the treatment note but then address all patient problems in the progress note.

When writing the Assessment section of the progress note, summarize the patient's status toward the goals set on the initial documentation. In doing so, indicate if the goal is met, not met (ongoing), or discontinued. Also, describe progress made toward the established goals. For example, indicate whether the patient is progressing toward goals that have not yet been met. Use the Assessment section of the progress note to justify progress that is faster or slower than what was initially expected, to link ongoing impairment to function, to highlight any new issue(s) interfering with the intervention, and to provide a rationale for discontinuing a goal(s). Use this area to document anything that helps justify ongoing services by giving a very clear picture (in terms others understand) of the patient's progress, ongoing problems and complications, and need for further skilled intervention. Also, include the patient's potential for further improvement. Finally, avoid general phrases such as, "The patient tolerated the treatment well."[3] The following examples are typical comments documented in the Assessment section of a treatment note or progress report.

1. Treatment and progress note examples:
   a. AROM [active range of motion] knee flexion increased 15 degrees after treatment.
   b. Pain decreased from 6/10 to 2/10 after treatment.
   c. Gait speed improved 0.2 m/s since yesterday.
   d. Patient's rate of perceived exertion after treatment today was 11; this is improved from yesterday when the rate of perceived exertion was 13.
   e. Patient was able to ambulate to and from the bathroom (~40') with minimal assist and cane today. This is improved from last treatment when he required a standard walker and moderate assist.

2. Progress note examples:
   a. Patient has met all established short-term goals and is progressing toward the long-term goals set on the initial documentation.
   b. Patient has achieved goals 1 to 3. Goals 4 and 5 are ongoing.
   c. Patient has met goals for transfers and bed mobility. Still needs to work on increasing strength in the lower extremity to prevent the knee from buckling during gait and increase independence in this area.
   d. Overall, the patient has made good progress toward goals; she is demonstrating a significant reduction in limb volume post-therapy and improved range of motion.
   e. Patient's progress has been slower than what was originally expected because of transportation issues and unexpected illness that have prevented her from attending regular therapy sessions.

Assessing Change

When assessing the patient for change, one should consider the measurement properties of the various instruments used during the initial examination. Measurement properties that are of particular value when assessing change include "normal" values or scores, degree of error associated with the tests and measures (eg, the standard error of the measurement [SEM]), and the clinical utility, such as the minimal detectable change (MDC) and the instrument's minimal clinically important difference (MCID) (see Chapter 9). For example, there are normal values associated with range of motion measures, blood pressure, and some patient questionnaires or functional assessments. When assessing and describing a patient's status, document whether a particular measurement falls into the "normal" range. In some cases, it may be necessary to

document why a patient's measurements have not returned to the normal value(s).

Familiarity with the degree of error associated with instruments used clinically will also help in assessing change. One common measurement of error found in the literature is the SEM.[4] The SEM is the *amount of error* associated with repeated measurements of the same patient.[4] The value of the SEM gives the amount of error in the same units as the original test or measure (eg, the SEM for goniometry would be given in degrees).[5,6] There are SEMs associated with single measures as well as with change scores. This is important for the therapist to consider when determining the patient's progress. Knowledge of the amount of error associated with a test or measure will help determine whether true change occurred or if patient change was due merely to error associated with repeated measurements. Let us look at an example from the literature. The authors of a 2006 study published in *Physical Therapy* reported the SEM for measuring gait speed measured on a GaitMat II.[7] The SEM for the participant's normal gait speed was 0.04 m/s and 0.05 m/s for faster speeds. Any change between the baseline and postintervention speed below the SEM may be indicative of measurement error, rather than true change due to treatment.

Let us apply these results to a patient in a clinical situation. A patient's gait speed at the initial encounter was 0.82 m/s. After a 4-week physical therapy intervention program, the patient's gait speed was 0.85 m/s, a difference of 0.03 m/s. In this case, yes, the patient has shown a change, and a clinician may be inclined to document an improvement in gait speed. However, given the amount of error associated with the measure, the change may be due to measurement error rather than true improvement in speed. Hence, a clinician should not conclude that the patient has made clinically meaningful progress.

After continuing the program for another 2 weeks, the patient's gait speed is reassessed. This time it is 0.92 m/s, a difference of 0.10 m/s since the initial visit. In this case, the clinician could conclude there has been a change outside the margin of error.

Familiarity with the SEM helps clinicians in making decisions with individual patients, allowing them to compare the patient's score or change score(s) to the degree of error associated with the test or measure.

In considering patient change, the clinician may also compare the patient's change score with the MDC of the instrument, much like he or she would compare against the SEM. However, the MDC is usually somewhat more conservative than the SEM, meaning the patient would usually have to change more to exceed the MDC than the SEM. Many researchers are investigating the MDC associated with clinical tests and measures. However, this has not always been the case, and the MDC is not known for many instruments we use clinically.

Another valuable estimate to help assess clinical change is the MCID. The MCID is used much like the SEM and

MDC previously described in that the patient's change scores are compared with the MCID. However, it is important to realize that the MCID is an estimate, and, like the MDC, we do not know the MCID for all tests and measures used in physical therapy.[7]

More research is needed to determine how values such as the SEM, MDC, and MCID can be generalized to patients in a clinical setting. Nevertheless, values identified in the literature provide a starting point for clinicians assessing change using an evidence-based approach. Understanding normal values, the SEM, MDC, and MCID provide us with benchmarks to not only establish goals for a patient but also to summarize meaningful patient change throughout the episode of care.

Plan

In the Plan section of a treatment or progress note, include any new skilled activities or interventions that are planned to address the patient's physical therapy problems. Use the plan to emphasize the progressive nature of the physical therapy services and the episode of care. For example, document the plan to progress the patient to a less supportive assistive device during gait as the patient's balance improves, or document the plan to advance a patient from range of motion to strengthening exercises. Any time new interventions are added or listed in the plan, provide a justification or explanation to show medical necessity. Make modifications to the previous plan of care including any changes to the patient's current intervention(s) or changes in the amount, frequency, or duration of services. In most cases, use the progress note, rather than the treatment note, to make significant changes to the plan of care.

When writing the plan, detailed and specific information is imperative. Clearly state the activities that will occur during upcoming sessions. It is also a good habit to regularly restate the amount, frequency, and duration of physical therapy sessions even if they are unchanged. Generally, avoid the frequent use of statements such as "Continue per plan of care." Repetitive, general entries would require a reviewer to search for the initial documentation in order to locate the current plan, and each note should act as a stand-alone document. The following statements would be appropriate for the Plan section of an interim note:

- Increase weight on terminal knee extensions on the next visit to further increase strengthening.
- Attempt gait with straight cane next session to improve independence.
- Try use of supine stander during the next session to promote weight bearing and upright posture during functional activities.
- Instruct patient's husband in guarding the patient on the stairs in the next session.

- Continue with treatment 2 times a day for the next 3 to 5 days at which point the patient is scheduled for discharge to an inpatient rehabilitation facility.
- Plan to continue with skilled care to instruct the patient and family in safe strengthening and range of motion exercises and to train patient's husband in the use of the Hoyer lift.

Timing Interim Notes

Documentation is required for every patient visit or encounter.[1] The frequency in which progress notes are written is dependent on the patient's rate of progress, the frequency of therapy sessions, the setting in which physical therapy is being provided, the policies and procedures of the facility, and the requirements set forth by regulating agencies and third-party payers. For example, in an outpatient setting, the Centers for Medicare & Medicaid Services requires a progress note, or report, every 10 treatment sessions.[8] In home health, reassessments and progress reports are also required every 30 days or by the 14th visit. Should services go beyond 14 visits, there must be another reassessment by the 20th visit.[9]

In general, progress notes are written more often when the patient's progress toward the stated goals occurs rapidly. In some situations, each treatment note serves as a progress note. For example, a patient in an acute care setting is recovering from a surgical procedure and significant improvements are seen daily; therefore, the physical therapist chooses to write a progress note daily to demonstrate this progress. Alternatively, within an inpatient rehabilitation setting, progress notes may be written on a weekly basis in order to report at team conferences, and in a long-term care setting progress notes may be written on a monthly basis. In practice areas that are not bound by policy or regulation to a particular time frame, progress note frequency mirrors the time frame for the established goals but, at minimum, should occur monthly.

RE-EVALUATIONS

Although therapists perform some aspects of re-examination and re-evaluation at each patient encounter, there are times when formal re-evaluations should occur. Formal re-evaluations are required when there has been *any significant change in the patient's status warranting a change in the plan of care*.[8] In addition, re-evaluation timing may occur as dictated by state law or facility policy. Recall from Chapter 4 that formal re-evaluations are different from regular reassessments. Re-evaluations have a separate billing code, whereas regular reassessments are part of the typical episode of care. Even though a re-evaluation has a separate billing code, there are stipulations as to whether it will be reimbursed. For example, the Centers for Medicare

& Medicaid Services guidelines indicate that reimbursement for a physical therapy re-evaluation requires a significant change in the patient's status that warrants a change in the plan of care (eg, a hospitalization or onset of a new or secondary diagnosis).[8] It is important to be familiar with third-party payer reimbursement guidelines prior to using certain billing codes such as physical therapy re-evaluation.

The documentation of a formal re-evaluation includes the same structure and elements described for the initial documentation and for a progress report. However, the emphasis in a re-evaluation is on data that are new or different. The Assessment section clearly describes patient changes that have occurred, goals that have been met, new goals, adaptations to the plan of care (goals, interventions, and frequency or duration of care), and the patient's continued need for skilled services. All changes to the plan of care are justified by evidence provided within the Subjective and Objective sections of the note.

LETTERS

A physical therapist at times needs to write letters to various individuals involved in the health care of the patient/client. In any setting, as a professional courtesy, the therapist will write letters to physicians of patients they are treating to provide a status update. This can happen at the onset of physical therapy services following the initial examination, intermittently throughout the episode of care, and/or at discharge. It is also beneficial for the therapist to communicate to a patient's physician regarding physical therapy interventions provided, even if the patient has sought physical therapy via direct access. Communicating in this way helps to build mutual respect between health care providers and, in turn, helps to facilitate the patient's overall health care.

When writing a letter to a physician, clearly and concisely tailor the information to address the areas in which the physician is most likely concerned or interested. Include a brief introduction and statement giving the patient information. Provide relevant subjective comments, objective findings, present problems, your overall impression, and your plan. Finally, as a courtesy, thank the physician for the referral (Example 10-1). Occasionally, physical therapists will create form letters and templates to facilitate the letter-writing process, and electronic documentation software often includes standard letters and forms to physicians that are populated with data from a previous progress or treatment note. Case managers and third-party payers may also request similar letters. Information provided in these types of letters is tailored to address the questions and concerns of the individual requesting the information. Keep a copy of any such written communication in the patient's physical therapy record.

Example 10-1. Letter to a Physician

Dear Dr. Smith,

I am writing to provide an update on your pt. Richard Jones (DOB: 3/3/1936), whom you referred to physical therapy for treatment following a (R) ankle fracture.

At this time (8 weeks post-fracture), he reports pain as 3/10 and notes improved function in the home and community. He has resumed independent ADLs and some home tasks. His AROM for DF is 10°, PF is 50°, inversion is 20°, and eversion is 5°. Strength is 4/5 throughout, and he is able to ambulate full weight bearing without an assistive device. His balance is fair and he is independent with all mobility on level surfaces.

He continues to have difficulty on uneven surfaces including ambulation on uneven ground. This is a problem since he works as a farmer. I would like to continue treatment 1 to 2 times weekly to progress strength, proprioception, higher level balance activities, and ankle strategies to improve ambulation on all surfaces. Please contact me at ###-###-#### if you have any questions or want to discuss this pt. further. Thank you for this referral, and I look forward to continuing to work with him.

Respectfully,

Sue Smith, DPT

SUMMARY

Interim notes include (1) treatment or daily notes that serve as a record of care provided and billed for that day of service using skilled terminology, (2) progress notes that justify ongoing services, and (3) re-evaluations that are done after a change in patient status. Interim documentation may also include letters and communication notes to other individuals involved with the patient when needed.

For treatment or daily notes, the clinician providing the intervention (ie, the physical therapist or the physical therapist assistant) completes the documentation. If more than one therapist or assistant treats a patient in a single session, then both individuals should authenticate, or sign, the documentation. Within this interim documentation, the physical therapist is solely responsible for modifying the plan of care, interpreting new orders, performing regular reassessments and formal re-evaluations, and writing the Assessment and Plan sections of the progress notes. A physical therapist assistant can write treatment notes and, where allowed by law, may write the Assessment and Plan sections of a treatment note. Within this documentation, a physical therapist assistant can document a need for changes to the plan of care, but it is the sole responsibility of the physical therapist to follow-up with the reassessment and record changes to the plan of care.

Interim notes are written in a manner to show consistency with the initial documentation to tell a story of the patient's episode of care. Interim notes reflect disablement concepts, clinical problem solving, and skilled care provided. Each note serves as evidence that will ultimately justify the patient's care.

REVIEW QUESTIONS

1. List the different types of interim notes. What is the purpose of each?

2. Compare and contrast a treatment note and a progress note. In your discussion, include the purpose of each and the contents of each.

3. Is a summary of patient progress a requirement for a treatment note or a progress note? Who decides the amount of progress summarized in a treatment note?

4. What information should be included in the Objective section of a treatment or progress note?

5. In what type of note are the patient's goals addressed and updated?

6. What information is required for documenting an intervention?

7. When and where should the justification for integrating a new intervention be provided in the documentation?

8. Compare and contrast the roles of the physical therapist and physical therapist assistant regarding interim documentation.

9. How is a re-evaluation different from a regular reassessment?

10. Of the following, which can be billed to the patient using a separate billing code: ongoing weekly assessment, a formal reassessment, and/or a formal re-evaluation?

APPLICATION EXERCISES

1. Write the following information in a more clear, concise manner as it would appear in the medical record. Replace the percentage of assistance provided with min, mod, or max assist where appropriate.

   a. You are working with a patient in an outpatient clinic with a diagnosis of right bicipital tendonitis. She tells you she has been working on the home exercises, and overall her arm is feeling much better. She reports improvements in dressing and fixing her hair. She reports her current pain to be 3/10 on a verbal pain scale. She says she has trouble reaching into overhead cabinets and shelves. Her treatment consisted of phonophoresis over the anterior shoulder for 8 minutes, 50% duty cycle with the intensity set at 1.5 w/cm^2. This was followed by active scapular retraction and protraction done in standing, active prone horizontal abduction, and standing external rotation done with a yellow exercise band for 2 sets of 10 repetitions with verbal and tactile cues for arm positioning. She also received manual therapy including grades 2 and 3 anteroposterior and inferior glenohumeral joint mobilizations to improve joint movement and decrease pain. The total exercise session lasted 30 minutes.

   b. You are working with an inpatient with Guillain-Barré syndrome. He reports he is doing better today with much less fatigue after the session yesterday. His therapeutic exercise consisted of ankle pumps, active hip abduction, heel slides, bridging, and knee extension at the edge of the mat (3 sets of 10 repetitions). After the exercises, you worked on functional training including transfers from the bed to and from the wheelchair using a stand pivot transfer. The patient required ~30% assistance from 1 therapist, although you did have to block his knees because of quadriceps weakness. At the end of the session, the patient required 60% assist to transfer back to bed because of mild fatigue. He positioned himself in bed with verbal cues and use of the side rails for assist to scoot. His ability to transfer has not improved in the last week. The plan is to work on gait training in the afternoon session.

   c. You are working with an elderly woman in the acute care setting who has suffered a right CVA 3 days ago. The patient is cooperative and complains of lack of mobility and function. You perform passive and active assistive range of motion on her left upper and lower extremities using facilitation techniques to promote active movement. The patient was not showing signs of abnormal tone or reflex development. You performed 30 repetitions for the upper and lower extremities. You also provided manual resistance for the right upper and lower extremities for 30 repetitions. You provided stretching to the left heel cords to increase joint range of motion to allow normal stance. The stretch was performed 5 times, holding for 30 seconds each time. The patient transferred out of bed with minimal assist of 1 to the wheelchair with stabilization for her left knee and trunk support. She ambulated twice in the parallel bars 8 feet with right upper extremity support. She required minimal assist of 1 for trunk support and moderate assist of 1 at the left lower extremity for swing, placement of the foot, and knee stabilization. The plan is for discharge in the next 1 to 2 days to inpatient rehabilitation. Your more immediate plan is to work with her twice daily on range of motion and mobility skills until discharge.

d. You are working with a patient 3 days status post–right total knee replacement in the therapy gym. Pain rating is 6/10. States she has rheumatoid arthritis (RA) and has difficulty getting moving. She states she wants to be discharged to home to live alone. She has noticeable swelling and limited range of motion in the knee and ankle. Active range of motion in the right knee measure 5 to 65 degrees. She transfers wheelchair to and from the mat with you providing 30% assistance because of her left lower extremity weakness and difficulty standing. She transferred sit to and from supine with you performing 50% assistance because of her inability to lift the right leg onto the mat table. She performed 2 sets of 10 repetitions of the total knee exercises and ambulated 50 feet, twice with a standard walker, putting only 50% of her body weight on the involved extremity. She required assistance for sequencing the walker and her steps to allow unweighting the involved extremity. She received ice for 15 minutes to her knee. You suspect her limited mobility and the fact she lives alone will require her to remain an inpatient longer than normal. You also suspect the RA may be limiting her progress. You will plan to continue with increasing ROM and independence with mobility until d/c and recommend a short-term post–acute care placement until independence improves.

e. You are working with a patient recently hospitalized for pneumonia, mild congestive heart failure and dementia, and lower extremity weakness. She tells you she is looking forward to going home where she lives alone. She complains of some difficulty breathing during the session. She is using oxygen provided by a nasal cannula on 2 L. The patient walked 150' where she required contact guard assist and monitoring because of her shortness of breath. You are monitoring her respiratory rate (14 breaths/minute prior to ambulation and 20 after). You also monitored her oxygen saturation level (94% prior to treatment and 90% after). She also demonstrated swaying during gait and complains of dizziness when turning her head during ambulation. You feel she is not ready to go home alone and should have continued therapy after discharge because of balance and endurance issues. Your plan is to continue working on increasing endurance and balance twice daily and to work with case management on transfer to the hospital's skilled unit.

2. Using the initial documentation on pp. 29 to 30 (Chapter 4, Amputation) to make comparisons, rewrite the following information into a progress report.

a. The patient is now 2 weeks s/p right transtibial amputation and is still in the inpatient rehabilitation setting. He is continuing to complain of phantom pain (he rates at 4/10) and sensation from the right foot. It resolves if he "squeezes" his residual limb. You are planning to attend a team conference for him on the following day, so you decide to take some objective measurements. Right active range of motion is hip flexion 120 degrees, hip extension lacking 5 degrees, hip abduction 40 degrees, hip adduction 10 degrees, knee flexion 130 degrees, and knee extension lacking 5 degrees. Passive range of motion is right knee and hip extension 0 degrees. Strength in the right lower extremity for hip flexion is 4/5, extension 4/5 in side-lying position, abduction 4/5, knee extension 3+/5, and knee flexion 4/5 in the side-lying position. The patient cannot lay prone because of pulmonary problems and difficulty breathing when in this position. The incision is closed, and there is a pink scar present. There is no drainage and no signs or symptoms of infection. It is moderately adhered to the underlying tissue and hypersensitive to pressure. Residual limb girth is 40 cm at the right knee joint, 41 cm 2 inches below, and 42 cm 4 inches below. The patient can move and transfer in and out of bed independently to a bedside commode or chair. He can manage the wheelchair parts with verbal cueing. He propels the wheelchair 50' independently on level surfaces and carpet and then requires a rest. He can ambulate 75' with a standard walker with supervision ×1, and his balance is good. Assist is required because he fatigues quickly and needs cueing for sequencing the walker. The patient is independent with residual limb care and using the shrinker sock. You have also made initial contact with a prosthetist regarding this patient. He is planning on going home in 1 to 2 weeks. You also plan to continue with skilled intervention for safely progressing exercises and endurance to improve mobility and independence in the home and to work on pain and edema control to prepare the limb for prosthesis and increase standing and mobility activities.

b. The patient is now 10 weeks s/p right transtibial amputation and is being seen as an outpatient. He has been receiving treatment as an outpatient for the last 2 weeks when he received his prosthesis. His goals for the outpatient setting (to be met over the next 2 months) are as follows:

   i. Normal range of motion in the residual limb to allow independence with prosthesis and a normal, efficient gait pattern.

   ii. Strength of the right lower extremity will be 5/5 to promote independence with prosthesis and a normal, efficient gait pattern.

   iii. Tolerate 8 hours of continuous prosthetic use without skin breakdown.

    iv. The patient will demonstrate good balance as evidenced by a score < 14 seconds on the Timed Up and Go (TUG).

    v. Ambulate > 300 m on the 6-minute walk test.

    vi. Score > 35 on the Amputee Mobility Predictor (AMP).

  c. Use the following information to write a progress note for this patient. Assume you have been treating this patient since his inpatient stay. Use the data in Application Exercise 2a as a comparison. Convert strength descriptions to manual muscle test grades. Include short-term goals. The patient is continuing to complain of phantom pain and sensation from the right foot occasionally, but it has decreased to 2/10. He is reporting improvements in his home environment including ambulation with the crutches for short distances and ability to wear the prosthesis for 2 to 3 hours. Reports his grandson has been staying with him to provide assist and transportation to therapy. Right active range of motion is hip flexion 120 degrees, hip extension 10 degrees, hip abduction 40 degrees, hip adduction 10 degrees, knee flexion 140 degrees, and knee extension 0 degrees. Strength in the right LE hip flexion 4/5, extension 4+/5 in side-lying position, abduction 4+/5, knee extension 4+/5, and knee flexion 4+/5 in side-lying position. The incision is not adhered to the underlying tissue, and sensitivity has subsided. Residual limb girth is 40 cm at the knee joint, 39 cm 2 inches below, and 39 cm 4 inches below. He is independent with all wheelchair parts and transfer. He propels the wheelchair 500' independently on level surfaces and carpet. He can ambulate 150' with axillary crutches with supervision ×1 and good balance without the prosthesis. He requires minimal assist to don and doff the socket and secure the supracondylar cuff suspension. He ambulates 50' with the prosthesis on and with axillary crutches with minimal assist for advancing the prosthesis. He is ambulating with an abducted gait on the prosthetic side. His TUG score is 22 seconds. His AMP score is 32. You would like to begin stair training with the prosthesis and advancing his gait skills (curbs, ramps, etc). You

would like to see him twice weekly. His motivation is good, and you believe his potential to improve is good. You spend 10 minutes educating the patient on skin precautions after removing the prosthesis and 15 minutes on exercises where he requires facilitation and manual cueing for proper performance. Minimal detectable change for outcome measures in this population are 45 m for the 6-minute walk test, 3.6 seconds for the TUG, and 3.4 for the AMP.[10]

3. Use the initial documentation you created in Chapter 9 Application Exercise #5 (CVA) and create a progress note based on the following information. On the third day of treatment, the patient states he feels he is getting stronger and is looking forward to continuing his recovery. The patient and his wife stated they discussed inpatient rehabilitation placement with case manager. The patient's wife states she is concerned about how they will manage in the long run. She says their son and daughter-in-law can provide some assistance, but she will be the primary caregiver. He needed moderate assistance when scooting up and down and side to side in bed. He was able to roll to the right without any assistance and was safe with the activity. He required minimal assistance when rolling to the left. The patient still displays significant edema (girth 43.6 cm) in his right hand and forearm and reports he forgets to use his positioning devices in bed and in the wheelchair. He required minimal assistance to transfer supine to sit. He requires minimal assistance when performing a sit-to-stand transfer and moderate assistance with a stand pivot transfer from the therapy mat into the wheelchair. He ambulated with a quad cane with min (a) ×1 to support his trunk and assist with balance and mod (a) ×1 to advance and stabilize the right leg. He ambulated 20' ×2 and then required a rest break. He requires a rest break 4× in a 30-minute session. You tell him you will see him again in the afternoon to work on more therapeutic exercises and to ambulate. You educated the patient's wife regarding his need for supervision and constant verbal cues because he is impulsive and unsafe at times.

REFERENCES

1. American Physical Therapy Association. Physical therapy documentation of patient/client management. BOD G03-05-16-41. 2014. http://www.apta.org/uploadedFiles/APTAorg/About_Us/Policies/Practice/DocumentationPatientClientManagement.pdf#search=%22Physical%20Therapy%20Documentation%20of%20Patient%2fClient%20Management%22. Accessed 2019.

2. American Physical Therapy Association. *Guide to Physical Therapist Practice.* 2016. http://guidetoptpractice.apta.org/. Accessed April 18, 2018.

3. Clifton D. "Tolerated treatment well" may no longer be tolerated. *PT Magazine.* 1995;3:24.

4. MacDermid J, Stratford P. Applying evidence on outome mesaures to hand therapy practice. *J Hand Ther.* 2004;17:165-173.

5. Finch E, Brooks D, Stratford P, Mayo N. *Physical Rehabilitation Outcome Measures.* 2nd ed. Philadelphia, PA: Lippincott Williams and Wilkins; 2002.

6. Domholdt E. *Physical Therapy Research: Principles and Applications.* 2nd ed. Philadelphia, PA: WB Saunders; 2000.

7. Palombaro K, Craik R, Mangione K, Tomlinson J. Determining meaningful changes in gait speed after hip fracture. *Phys Ther.* 2006;86:809-816.

8. Centers for Medicare & Medicaid Services. Covered medical and other health services. *Medicare Benefit Policy Manual.* Publication 100-02. 2019. https://www.cms.gov/Regulations-and-Guidance/Guidance/Manuals/Downloads/bp102c15.pdf. Accessed May 3, 2019.

9. Centers for Medicare & Medicaid Services. Home health services. *Medicare Benefit Policy Manual.* Publication 100-02. http://www.cms.gov/Regulations-and-Guidance/Guidance/Manuals/Downloads/bp102c07.pdf. 2019.

10. Resnick L, Borgia M. Reliability and outcome measures for people with lower-limb amputations: distinguishing true change from error. *Phys Ther.* 2011;91:555-565.

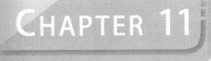

Patient Outcomes and Discharge Summaries

Rebecca S. McKnight, PT, MS and Mia L. Erickson, PT, EdD

CHAPTER OUTLINE

- Documenting Outcomes
  - The Discharge Summary
    - Subjective
    - Objective
    - Assessment
    - Plan
- Outcomes and Health Care Administration
- A Plan for Assessing Outcomes

CHAPTER OBJECTIVES

Upon completion of this chapter, the reader will be able to:

1. Define outcome
2. Recognize the importance of examining outcomes for cohorts and individual patients
3. Describe the benefits of using functional assessments as outcomes measures
4. Construct an appropriate discharge summary
5. Integrate measures of clinical change such as MDC and MCID in outcomes
6. Realize the use of functional assessments in quality initiatives
7. Describe the barriers associated with using functional assessments in outcomes data collection
8. Outline practical suggestions for establishing a clinical outcomes data collection process

Erickson ML, Utzman RR, McKnight RS.
Physical Therapy Documentation: From Examination to Outcome,
Third Edition (pp 109-116).
© 2020 Taylor & Francis Group.

KEY TERMS

cohort
functional assessment
outcome
outcomes assessment
outcomes research

KEY ABBREVIATIONS

MCID
MDC

Over the last decades, outcomes assessment and outcomes research have become mainstays in physical therapy practice, research, and policy making. A patient's outcome is the end result of his or her health care for a given injury, disease, or condition. The *Guide to Physical Therapist Practice* defines outcome as the "impact," or end result, of patient/client management.[1] There are many different ways to assess a patient's outcome. Physical therapists are often interested in examining the effects of the intervention provided, whether it is a procedural intervention, such as therapeutic exercise or a specific modality, or a nonprocedural intervention, such as patient education. There are many ways to examine the effects of our intervention. At the conclusion of the episode of care, a variety of factors, or outcome variables, may be analyzed such as the patient's pathology, impairments, functional status, risk reduction, overall health or wellness, or satisfaction, to name a few.[1] Additional outcome variables important to physical therapists as well as others involved in the patient's care include the quality and value of the health care provided,[2] especially with regard to the overall cost of the intervention(s) and the degree of improvement attained. Other outcome variables include things such as time lost from work, lost wages, return-to-work status, the number of visits or sessions, hospital readmission, and the total cost of treatment provided. When examining the effects of the intervention, it is important to remember the outcome is determined by patient factors, behavior, or status and not by provider behavior. For example, a physical therapist measuring outcomes attempts to determine the effectiveness of an intervention, so he measures the patient's functional performance, impairments, return to independent living, and societal integration following a traumatic injury. Measurements of provider actions, such as whether the therapist is tracking patient education, are not patient outcome indicators.[3]

A patient determines the effects of treatment based on things he or she cares most about, such as functional change and improved quality of life.[2] In the late 1980s, medical professionals, including rehabilitation professionals, began using functional assessment as a means for measuring outcome in order to capture things that matter most to patients.[2,4] Functional measures consider the patient's perspective of his or her abilities and overall well-being, and they provide a powerful assessment of patient change during the time the treatment was provided.[5] Functional assessments also help health care providers communicate the patient's functional status with others. The use of functional terminology provides insight into how the injury or illness affects the patient's day-to-day life in terms laypeople understand.[6] Without functional measures, "payers cannot understand us when we attempt to communicate."[5(p1)] However, the aforementioned benefits of functional assessment are not intended to indicate that impairment measures are not important. In fact, one should integrate both together because they are relevant to research, practice, and development of the profession's scientific body of knowledge.[6]

DOCUMENTING OUTCOMES

Physical therapists examine outcomes for cohorts or individual patients.[3,7] A cohort is a group of patients with a similar injury, diagnosis, or characteristics (eg, rotator cuff repair or traumatic brain injury). One way to assess outcomes for a cohort is to perform the same tests and measures on each group member at the same point in time. For example, a therapist examining the effectiveness of a balance and falls program might assess participants' fall risk prior to participation and again 4, 8, and 12 weeks after beginning participation. Additionally, one could perform the same measures at some point following program completion, such as 1 year after completing the program. Clinicians and researchers use measures in this manner to provide insight to program and treatment effectiveness. Data are used in program quality improvement, marketing materials, publications, and professional presentations.

Individual patient outcomes are considered throughout the episode of care. First, the therapist considers "an expected outcome" for every patient that is articulated through outcome, or discharge, goals. At each reassessment, the therapist considers and documents progress toward the outcome goals by comparing current and prior subjective and objective data. At the end of the episode of care, the physical therapist documents the patient's outcome, or end result, in a discharge summary. The following section describes components of a properly constructed discharge summary, and a documentation template for creating a discharge summary can be found in Table 11-1.

TABLE 11-1	
DISCHARGE SUMMARY TEMPLATE	
SUBJECTIVE	Provide patient/family/caregiver remarks regarding final status, improvement, independence, etc. Provide information regarding the benefits of treatment, improved daily living, performance of functional tasks. Provide status regarding chief complaints and functional problems identified in the initial documentation. Provide any other subjective information that gives insight to the patient's final status.
OBJECTIVE	Document results of relevant tests and measures that are consistent with initial, or prior, documentation. Document intervention(s) provided on the final day of service including patient-related instruction. Summarize the intervention(s) provided throughout the episode of care.
ASSESSMENT	Give the reason for discharge. Summarize the effects of the intervention(s) on impairment, function, risks, health and wellness, societal resources, or any other aims of the intervention(s). Summarize patient change using measures from the literature (eg, normal values, minimal detectable change, clinically important difference). Give the status toward the discharge or outcome goals set by the physical therapist. Describe any remaining issues, problems, or goals that have not been met and provide a rationale. Describe any comorbidity or factor(s) complicating the episode of care.
PLAN	List any patient, provider, family member, or caregiver activity that will take place following the final session. Give the discharge destination (eg, inpatient rehabilitation) or participation status (eg, return to work).

The Discharge Summary

Subjective

The discharge summary includes the final subjective remarks given in a manner similar to the initial documentation. It includes comments that will allow direct comparisons between the initial or prior documentation and the final documentation in the areas of patient complaints, concerns, and goals. It includes the patient's or family members' remarks regarding the patient's overall improvement, the current functional status, and any changes brought on by the intervention(s). The discharge summary also provides comments given by the patient, family, or caregiver describing functional improvements brought on by the reduction of impairments (Example 11-1).

Objective

In addition to the final subjective status, the discharge documentation includes the results of objective tests and measures used to make comparisons between initial, prior, and current impairments and functional status. It includes new tests and measures when needed, such as strength or muscle testing, that were not appropriate at the initial visit because of surgical precautions. All tests and measures accurately reflect the patient's status at the conclusion of the episode of care. In the Objective section of the discharge summary, the physical therapist summarizes the skilled care provided throughout the episode to give a final justification for why it was medically necessary. This is not an "all inclusive" list but rather a summary describing important components of care provided. The final documentation also includes a list of skilled treatment provided and billed on the final day of service. Subheadings or section headers are used to differentiate between services provided during the final encounter and those provided in other sessions (Example 11-2).

However, there may be times when a final reassessment is not performed, such as when the patient is discharged by the physician or the patient stops coming to therapy. In

Example 11-1. Discharge Subjective

Pt. reports he is now able to get in and out of bed independently and no longer requires assist from wife.

Pt. reports that all rehabilitation goals are met.

Pt. states that stretching brought on improved knee ROM and allows improvement in ascending and descending stairs.

Pt.'s daughter indicated that family training helped her in increasing safety during transferring the pt. and that she can do it without difficulty.

Pt. stated that balance training has helped her to feel more "steady," and she reports a decrease in the amount of "stumbling" over the last 3 months.

Example 11-2. Interventions Documented at Discharge

Today's treatment: 15 minutes of therapeutic activities on the mat working on LE strength to facilitate the quads, gluts, and hip abductors; also included sit-to-stand transfers to increase performance and strength. Pt. was instructed in and performed final home exercises without difficulty (attached handout) for 15 minutes. Pt.'s daughter was instructed in car transfers and

methods to safely assist the pt. for 15 minutes. Total time today 45 minutes.

Summary of episode of care: Pt.'s episode of care has included various activities to improve strength of the LEs to improve mobility in/out of bed and during ambulation, balance training to decrease her fall risk, and functional training to facilitate independent living.

Example 11-3. No Discharge Reassessment

The pt. did not return for her final visit; objective measurements show status at the time of the last visit, 1 week ago.

Pt. discharged from unit suddenly, and formal discharge assessment was not performed. Objective measures are from last session, 5/15/18.

these cases, the physical therapist incorporates data from the previous measurements and provides the date it was recorded (Example 11-3).

Assessment

The physical therapist documents the Assessment and Plan sections of the discharge summary. In the Assessment section, he or she provides a reason for the patient's discharge and a summary of meaningful patient change that occurred as a result of the episode of care. There are many reasons why patients are discharged from physical therapy services. Those include, but are not limited to, all established goals were met, the patient or family/caregiver declined further intervention, or the patient became unable to participate. In this section, the therapist summarizes specific changes occurring in the patient's initial pathology, impairments, function, risk, overall health or wellness, or societal resources (eg, assistance needed) since the

onset of treatment (Table 11-2).[1] The physical therapist uses his or her knowledge of the scientific evidence to determine whether clinically significant, meaningful changes occurred and describes data using the evidence if appropriate. This aids in describing the effects of the intervention on impairment reduction and functional improvement. Also, the therapist provides the patient's status toward the outcome goals (eg, goal met, goal ongoing, progress made, or goal discontinued) and overall satisfaction with the improvement. In addition, the final documentation includes any remaining issues, problems, or goals that have not been achieved and the reason(s), such as a comorbidity or complication (Examples 11-4 and 11-5).

Plan

In the Plan section of the discharge documentation, the physical therapist provides a list of anything that will take place following the final session with the patient. Depending on the patient, the length and contents of this section will vary. Examples of information include any plans for intervention at another setting (eg, inpatient rehabilitation, home health care, or outpatient therapy), independent or maintenance intervention through a home program, obtaining assistive or adaptive equipment, and transition into participation such as returning to work, school, recreation, or community activities. The physical therapist documents any plans for working toward goals that have not been met, referring the patient to another provider or individual who will assist the patient, and communicating with other individuals regarding the patient's care or status (Examples 11-6 and 11-7).

TABLE 11-2
DOMAINS ADDRESSED DURING PHYSICAL THERAPY INTERVENTIONS AND SAMPLE DOCUMENTATION OF PATIENT STATUS AT DISCHARGE

IF YOUR INTERVENTION ADDRESSES:	SAMPLE DOCUMENTATION
Pathology	Patient no longer showing signs or symptoms of complex regional pain syndrome Patient no longer showing signs or symptoms of patellar tendinitis
Impairment	Range of motion of the (L) shoulder is WNL in all planes and equal to the (R) Strength (L) elbow is 5/5 in all directions
Activity limitation	Patient can ascend and descend stairs independently Patient can perform all transfers without limitation
Participation restriction	Patient now able to participate in all school-related activities without limitation Patient now safe with unlimited community ambulation
Risk reduction and prevention	Patient now independent with all lifting tasks and shows good body mechanics
Health, wellness, and fitness	Patient is independent with fitness program
Societal resources	Patient is independent in use of public transportation
Patient satisfaction	Patient is pleased with her status and feels that she can discontinue therapy

Example 11-4. Discharge Assessment 1

The pt. has met all goals for physical therapy except for return to work; however, his case manager is working on a placement for him to begin right away. The interventions have helped in increasing mobility, strength, and functional restoration. His wrist mobility is now WNL. He also demonstrated a significant improvement (> 50#) in grip strength, and it is now 80% of his opposite side. His functional assessment decreased from 85% to 5%, suggesting minimal to no disability. He is also independent with his home program.

Example 11-5. Discharge Assessment 2

The pt. has met all goals established and has demonstrated significant improvement since the initial visit. Following exercises and functional training, she now demonstrates the ability to move in and out of bed independently, ambulates household distances independently and safely with a standard walker, and ascends and descend stairs with minimal supervision provided by her husband. She performs all exercises independently without cueing. Today her husband demonstrated independence with the car transfer, and all questions were answered. Pt. will still need to work on her goal of independent community ambulation.

> ## Example 11-6. Plan from Discharge Note 1
>
> Pt. will be discharged from physical therapy to an independent home exercise program and will return to work at his prior level of employment. He will call if questions arise.

> ## Example 11-7. Plan from Discharge Note 2
>
> Pt. will continue with therapy services through outpatient day program here at the hospital. He will receive further intervention for planning for community integration, such as identifying appropriate employment. Will speak with case manager about physical capabilities to assist with this transition.

OUTCOMES AND HEALTH CARE ADMINISTRATION

Clinicians, managers, and payers alike are interested in patients' outcome data from an administrative perspective. For example, functional measures have become associated with measuring health care quality and provider performance.[8] Administrators use data to assess clinic-wide or individual provider credibility and accountability, inform decision making about specific interventions or programs, and improve program quality. Additionally, the Centers for Medicare & Medicaid Services is including functional assessments as a quality indicator in the Physician Quality Reporting System program.[9]

However, there are considerations with using functional assessments to determine quality. First, clinicians should implement tests and measures repeatedly, so quality assessment is based on the patient's change over time rather than on a single evaluation.[10] Also, one must realize longer periods of observation minimize the connection between the outcome(s) and the care provided. Extraneous factors affecting both patients and providers begin weighing more heavily as time goes on, making it more difficult to draw conclusions about the quality of providers and the care rendered.[10] Patient factors such as disease progression, comorbidities, cointerventions, adherence, motivation, socioeconomic status, education level, and payer source may affect outcome data either positively or negatively. Provider and organizational factors such as documentation procedures, measurement variability between providers, differing intervention strategies, time allotment, data storage, and types of measurements selected to determine outcome also

influence data. In addition, "from both a conceptual and methodological perspective, outcomes assessment must take into account all of the services received from all providers involved in the patient care process."[11(pp111-112)] This is important in multidisciplinary settings such as inpatient rehabilitation, where a patient may be receiving multiple services such as physical therapy, occupational therapy, speech therapy, neuropsychology, nutritional services, and others. Clinicians must consider these issues because "collecting and reporting bad data simply because it is available does nothing to aid in informed decision making or maximization of outcome effect."[3(p302)]

A PLAN FOR ASSESSING OUTCOMES

Prior to establishing an outcomes measurement plan, determine (1) its purpose, (2) the source of data, (3) the procedures and/or individual(s) responsible for data collection, and (4) the individual(s) responsible for storing and analyzing data. Address both practical and logistical factors by asking who, what, where, when, why, and how. The following are examples[11]:

1. Who will collect the data?
   a. Examples: The physical therapist during the initial visit and the office staff during initial paperwork
2. What kind of data/measurements will be collected?
   a. Examples: Impairments, function, self-report questionnaires, global health-related quality of life questionnaires, and disease-specific questionnaires
3. Are measurements reliable and valid? What is the associated error, minimal detectable change (MDC), or minimal clinically important difference (MCID)?
4. What are the hallmarks of a good or bad outcome?
5. Where will data be collected?
   a. Examples: Clinic or hospital, paper or electronic, or completion at home
6. When will data be collected?
   a. Examples: Initial visit, 4 weeks, or after × number of visits
7. Why will the data be collected?
   a. Examples: How will the data be used? What is the purpose? To whom will the data be provided?
8. How will data be collected?
   a. Examples: Procedures for ongoing data collection or tracking when data need to be collected

Regardless of the benefits that arise from good data collection and reporting, barriers exist.[3] Barriers include personnel resistance to implementing new data collection procedures, time needed for performing, documenting, storing, retrieving, analyzing, and reporting data, and the need for consistency in patient coding (ie, the *International Classification of Diseases, Tenth Revision*) to facilitate data retrieval. In addition, there may be direct and indirect costs associated with new equipment, instruments, personnel, or training. Another consideration is whether to use a computerized outcomes management software package. These can be expensive because of the associated costs of hardware, software, upgrades, and report generation.

SUMMARY

Functional assessment as a means of outcome data collection is becoming more widespread, and the use of patient questionnaires and performance measures is growing. Whether data are collected for groups or individual patients, in implementing these measures, a clinician needs to identify valid instruments reflecting the aspects of health he or she is interested in measuring as well as their associated measurement properties. These can be used to establish goals or benchmarks as well as to describe meaningful patient change. There are many uses for outcome data, and clinicians need to consider the entire process when implementing.

REVIEW QUESTIONS

1. In your own words, define outcome.
2. What are the benefits of assessing patient function?
3. List the components of a discharge summary.
4. How are disablement concepts integrated into a discharge summary?
5. Why is consistency between the initial, subsequent (or interim), and discharge documentation important?
6. Give 3 different patient cohorts. Provide examples of medical record data that would be useful in examining treatment effectiveness for these groups.
7. What is the importance of knowing the standard error of the measurement when assessing a patient's outcome? How can the MDC and MCID be used in assessing outcome?
8. How can outcomes assessments be used in quality initiatives?
9. Describe some barriers associated with outcomes data collection.

APPLICATION EXERCISES

1. Identify one functional outcome test or measure for each of the following settings. Research its measurement properties. Give the following measurement properties: standard error of the measurement, MDC, and MCID. Determine if it is generic or disease (body-part) specific. Determine the administration technique (ie, patient performance or self-report).

   a. Acute care setting
   b. Inpatient rehabilitation unit
      i. Neurologic disorder
      ii. Musculoskeletal disorder
   c. Skilled nursing unit
   d. Home health
   e. Outpatient adult ambulatory clinic
      i. Upper extremity
      ii. Lower extremity
      iii. Spine
      iv. General
   f. Cardiopulmonary patient (Dx: COPD) in home health
   g. Pediatric outpatient clinic—neurologic disorders
   h. Pediatric outpatient clinic—musculoskeletal disorders
   i. Pediatric school setting—ages 5 to 9 years old
   j. Early intervention (birth to 3 years old)

2. Identify a setting (like the ones listed in Exercise 1) and a common diagnosis seen in that particular setting. Determine how you could go about implementing an outcomes assessment program for those patients.

3. Identify one clinician in your area and interview him or her regarding the use of outcomes assessment tools in the clinical setting. What instruments does he or she use? How are they used (eg, when is it administered, who administers it, how is it stored, etc)? How has it influenced his or her practice? How has it influenced reimbursement? How is it incorporated into his or her documentation?

4. Using the initial documentation from Chapter 9, complete a discharge summary using the information here.

One week later after the initial examination, the patient is being discharged to inpatient rehabilitation. You work with him just prior to his discharge. He states he has made a lot of recovery in 1 week. During the discharge examination, you identify the following. He continues to have pitting edema in the (R) hand and forearm and tends to keep his (R) UE in a dependent position. He maintains the extremity in the appropriate position with verbal cueing. The figure 8 hand girth is (R) 53.5 cm. His sensation is diminished to light touch, deep pressure localization, proprioception, and kinesthesia through the (R) UE and LE. Muscle tone shows a grade of 0 on the upper extremities and 1 on the lower extremities using the Modified Ashworth Scale. At the (R) shoulder, there is a 1 finger width sulcus at the GH joint. Muscle strength in the shoulder, elbow, and wrist remain 2−/5 and finger flexion is 1/5. Hip strength is 3/5 for flexion and extension and 3−/5 for abduction, adduction, internal rotation, and external rotation. Knee flexion is 3−/5 and extension is 3−/5. Ankle strength is 2−/5 for dorsiflexion and plantarflexion. He is able to stand without physical assistance or UE support at a quad cane with supervision with erect posture. During his therapy session today, the patient required minimal assistance of 1 with scooting up, down, and side-to-side. He was independent with rolling to the right and required minimal assist of 1 to roll to the left and for supine-to-sit transfers. He requires supervision when performing a sit-to-stand transfer and stand pivot transfer from the bed into the wheelchair for safety. He ambulated with a quad cane with min (a) ×1 to support his trunk and assist with balance and min (a) ×1 to advance and stabilize the right leg. He ambulated 35' × 2 and then required a rest break. He requires 2 rest breaks in a 30-minute session. He continues to be impulsive and a safety risk. He still plans to ultimately go home and live with his wife.

REFERENCES

1. American Physical Therapy Associaiton. *Guide to Physical Therapist Practice*. 2016. http://guidetoptpractice.apta.org/. Accessed April 18, 2018.
2. Agency for Healthcare Research and Quality. Outcomes research (fact sheet). AHRQ Publication 00-P011. http://www.ahrq.gov/clinic/outfact.htm. Accessed.
3. Ingersoll G. Generating evidence through outcomes management. In: Melnyk B, Fineout-Overholt E, eds. *Evidence-Based Practice in Nursing and Healthcare: A Guide to Best Practice*. Philadelphia, PA: Lippincott Williams & Wilkins; 2005:299-332.
4. Granger C. Quality and outcome measures for rehabilitation programs. https://emedicine.medscape.com/article/317865-overview. Published 2019. Accessed May 4, 2019.
5. Hart D. What should you expect from the study of clinical outcomes? *J Orthop Sports Phys Ther*. 1998;28:1-2.
6. Jette A. Outcomes research: shifting the dominant research paradigm in physical therapy. *Phys Ther*. 1995;75:965-970.
7. Finch E, Brooks D, Stratford P, Mayo N. *Physical Rehabilitation Outcome Measures*. 2nd ed. Philadelphia, PA: Lippincott Williams & Wilkins; 2002.
8. Resnik L, Liu D, Hart D, Mor V. Benchmarking physical therapy clinical performance: statistical methods to enhance internal validity when using observational data. *Phys Ther*. 2008:1078-1087.
9. Centers for Medicare & Medicaid Services. Quality measures. https://www.cms.gov/Medicare/Quality-Initiatives-Patient-Assessment-Instruments/QualityMeasures/index.html. Published 2019. Updated March 5, 2019. Accessed May 3, 2019.
10. Lohr K. Outcomes measurement: concepts and questions. *Inquiry*. 1988;25:37-50.
11. Wakefield D. Measuring health care outcomes: more work to do. *J Orthop Sports Phys Ther*. 1998;27:111-113.

CHAPTER 12

Documentation, Insurance, and Payment

Ralph R. Utzman, PT, MPH, PhD

CHAPTER OUTLINE

- Insurance Basics
  - Managed Care and Cost Containment
- More About Medicare
  - Part A
    - Acute Care Hospital Reimbursement
    - Inpatient Rehabilitation Facilities
    - Skilled Nursing Facilities and Subacute Care Units
    - Home Health Care
  - Part B
  - Part C
  - Part D
- Processes for Managing Reimbursement Claims
  - Before Care Is Delivered
  - During Patient Care
    - Diagnosis Coding
    - Coding for Procedures
  - Billing
  - Claims Denials and Appeals

Erickson ML, Utzman RR, McKnight RS.
Physical Therapy Documentation: From Examination to Outcome,
Third Edition (pp 117-130).
© 2020 Taylor & Francis Group.

CHAPTER OBJECTIVES

Upon completion of this chapter, the reader will be able to:

1. Describe how insurance protects patients from financial risk
2. List sources of funding for health insurance plans
3. Outline methods used by insurance companies to control costs
4. Define prospective payment
5. Compare different payment models: fee-for-service, payment per visit or per day, payment per episode, and capitation
6. List the 4 main "parts" of Medicare and state what types of services are covered by each.
7. Identify the payment methodology used by Medicare in the following settings: outpatient, acute care hospital, inpatient rehabilitation facility, skilled nursing facility, and home health.
8. Discuss the importance of gathering registration and insurance information prior to the initiation of care.
9. Name both the current and planned systems for coding patient diagnoses.
10. Name the system used to code for services and procedures.
11. Discuss how coding systems allow for transmission of billing claims from health care providers to insurers.
12. Discuss the importance of documentation for the prevention of claims denials.
13. Describe documentation strategies to prevent claims denials

KEY TERMS

Accountable Care Organization
advance beneficiary notice
bundling
capitation
Centers for Medicare & Medicaid Services
Current Procedural Terminology
copay
diagnosis-related groups
deductible
Explanation of Benefits
fee-for-service
fee schedule
International Classification
of Diseases, Tenth Revision
managed care
Medicaid
Medicare
Medicare administrative contractors
Medicare Post-Acute Care Transformation
(IMPACT) Act
Medicare Physician Fee Schedule
Merit-based Incentive Payment System
Outcome and Assessment Information Set
Overutilization
Patient-Driven Grouping Model
Patient-Driven Payment Model
Patient Protection and Affordable Care Act
(PPACA)
preauthorizaton
prospective payment system
relative value unit
value-based payment

KEY ABBREVIATIONS

ACO
CMS
CPT
DRG
ICD-10
IMPACT Act
IRF
MAC
MIPS
OASIS
PDPM
PPACA
RVU
SNF

Payment for physical therapist services is dependent on clear, concise, and accurate documentation. Depending on the care setting and payer source, third-party payers consider a combination of factors to determine payment, including patient diagnosis, severity of illness, functional status, treatment provided, and outcomes of care. This chapter introduces basic insurance concepts and current and emerging payment models for physical therapy care. Because of Medicare's importance in setting payment policy, the chapter also provides a brief background of Medicare. The chapter outlines the process for claims submission, including coding systems for diagnoses and procedures. Because insurance payment models are complex and evolving rapidly, the chapter focuses on basic concepts and trends rather than providing specific details. Links for additional information and suggestions for keeping current in your practice area are provided.

INSURANCE BASICS

Insurance provides a person with protection from financial risks. Most people do not have enough money in their savings accounts to purchase a new home if their house burns down or to buy a new car in case of an accident or theft. Homeowner and auto insurance help cover these costs. Likewise, health insurance protects people from financial catastrophe if they have an illness or an injury.

Insurance provides this financial protection by creating a pool of money that can be used to provide coverage for a large group of people. When a covered event (such as a fire, a car accident, or an illness) occurs, money from the pool is used to cover the necessary expenses. In the case of home and car insurance, most people pay regular premiums, which are added to the pool of money. In the case of health care insurance, most Americans do not directly pay the premiums that fund their health care insurance. For 49% percent of the US population, part or all of their health insurance premiums are paid by their employers as a benefit of employment.[1] Medicare and Medicaid are public, tax-funded programs that provide insurance coverage for older, retired adults and some younger people who do not have access to employer-sponsored insurance. Nearly 35% of the population is covered by Medicare and/or Medicaid.[1] About 7% of Americans pay for their own health insurance premiums. The remaining 9% has no health insurance.[1]

Traditionally, insurance plans have paid for health care using an indemnity model similar to car and home insurance. A patient with an indemnity plan would seek care from a health care provider and then pay for the care delivered. The patient would then seek reimbursement from the insurance company. In more contemporary indemnity plans, the health care provider submits the claim on the patient's behalf and is paid directly by the insurer.

The traditional indemnity model of insurance payment reimburses providers for every single procedure or service they provide. For a patient in the hospital, the insurance company would be billed for every aspirin, wound dressing, and therapy visit the patient receives. In this fee-for-service model, insurance companies assume the highest financial risk and least control compared with other payment models. Contemporary insurance plans that pay using a fee-for-service model will typically set or negotiate a fee schedule that specifies how much the plan will pay for each individual procedure.

Because the fee-for-service model is risky for insurers, they have developed various reimbursement models that bundle services together into more affordable packages. Consider the "combo meal" pricing strategy used by many fast-food restaurants. The combo meal bundles individual items together at a discounted price. In health care, services can be bundled in several ways. The most common strategies in physical therapy care are bundling by visit, by day, or by episode.

When care is bundled by visits, the insurer pays a set rate for each visit. The health care provider receives the same amount of payment per visit regardless of the number of services or products received during the visit. In inpatient settings, it makes more sense to bundle by day or per diem (ie, the insurer will pay a daily fee to the facility regardless of the services the patient receives each day). Payment can also be bundled by an entire episode of care. In this model, the provider receives a lump sum payment for an entire episode of care, such as a hospital stay. Regardless of the length of the episode of care and the intensity of the care provided, the provider or hospital receives the same lump sum payment. These models pose fewer financial risks for insurance companies than fee-for-service payment. Health care providers have more incentive to provide effective and efficient care to keep costs down. Bundled models are often called prospective payment systems because the amount of reimbursement is determined before the episode of care ends.

Managed Care and Cost Containment

Over the past several decades, the costs of health care in the United States have risen dramatically. Although there are many reasons for the rise in costs, our insurance system has been identified as a contributing factor. The administrative costs associated with managing and submitting insurance claims are high. Furthermore, insurance insulates both patients and health care providers from the costs of health care. Patients and providers make different choices than they would make if patients paid for health care out of their own pockets, leading to overutilization of services.[2] Managed care is one approach to slowing the rise in costs. In managed care plans, insurance companies have more control over the care delivered to patients. There are many different types of managed care plans, but all use a variety of cost-control mechanisms. These mechanisms are designed to influence the choices of patients and the practice behaviors of clinicians and health care facilities.

Managed care plans influence patient behavior through gatekeeping, cost sharing, or restricting choice. Gatekeeping involves requiring a referral from a primary care physician to see a specialist or to receive certain tests or therapeutic procedures. Cost sharing involves having the patient pay annual deductibles or copays for each visit. With a deductible, the patient is required to pay for a certain amount of care each year (eg, $1000) before the health insurance begins to pay. A copay is a fee that the patient pays at each visit. For example, a patient may have a $25 copay for each outpatient physical therapy visit. Managed care companies may restrict patient choice by requiring them to seek care from specific doctors, therapists, or hospitals that are members of the managed care network. Other plans may allow patients to seek care from out-of-network providers or facilities if they pay larger copays.

To control the behavior of clinicians, managed care plans develop employment or contractual arrangements with providers. Some health maintenance organizations hire all their health care providers, including physicians, as employees; these are called staff model health maintenance organizations. Independent practice associations or preferred provider organizations develop contractual agreements with physicians and other providers who agree to accept negotiated payment rates for delivering care. Managed care plans may also use case management processes to review care and approve payment for services to individual patients. For example, a managed care company may require a physical therapy plan of care to be reviewed for preauthorization before intervention can be provided. Some managed care companies will review documentation periodically during an episode of care to make sure care is being delivered appropriately and efficiently. They may also review payment claims and documentation after an episode of care is complete. If documentation does not demonstrate that appropriate care was provided, the managed care plan will deny reimbursement for part or all of the claim.

Managed care plans influence patient and clinician behavior, and thus costs of care, by placing limits and exclusions on care. For example, plans may exclude payment for certain patient diagnoses or treatments. Some plans will limit the number of outpatient therapy visits they will pay for per year. Others may limit the number of therapy procedures they will pay for per visit. Others will place a cap on the dollar amount they will reimburse for therapy per year. Finally, managed care companies can use different payment methodologies to encourage clinicians to limit unnecessary care.

Capitation is an example of an alternative payment model used by some managed care companies to control costs. In a capitation payment system, the health care provider agrees to provide care for a defined group of people for a set period of time. Capitation payment models pose lower financial risks to managed care companies because care is bundled for an entire group of people over a period of time. The health care provider receives the same amount of money regardless of how many people in the group need care or how the care is provided.

Managed care plans became very popular in the 1990s due to their potential to reduce health care costs and thus reduce insurance premiums paid by individuals, employers, and taxpayers. These various approaches achieved only modest success at slowing the rise in costs. In 2010, President Barack Obama signed the Patient Protection and Affordable Care Act (PPACA). This law established an extensive series of reforms for the US health care system. One portion of the PPACA promotes the development of value-based payment models that hold health care providers responsible for reducing costs while providing high-quality integrated care.[3] As a result, numerous Accountable Care Organizations (ACOs) have been developed since the PPACA was signed into law. Hospitals, health systems, and physician groups can develop ACOs, and physical therapists can be ACO participants. Each ACO is different, serving different parts of the population with different health needs. What they share is the goal of providing coordinated interprofessional services so that patients receive the right care, from the right provider, at the right time to optimize patient health and reduce waste. The program provides financial incentives for ACOs that can demonstrate cost savings while improving care quality (ie, increase value).[4,5] Currently, Medicare and Medicaid are leading the way by adopting value-based payment initiatives. Over time, strategies developed by ACOs that are proven to reduce costs while promoting quality will continue to be integrated into our health care system.

More About Medicare

Medicare is a social insurance program that was established in 1965 to provide health insurance coverage for Americans 65 years and older and for younger Americans with disabilities and end-stage renal disease.[6] Congress created the program by enacting Title XVIII of the Social Security Act. At the same time, Congress passed Title XVII, which created Medicaid to provide insurance coverage for low-income citizens who are younger than 65 years.[7] These laws created a federal agency, now known as the Centers for Medicare & Medicaid services (CMS), to oversee both programs. To administer the Medicare program, CMS contracts with regional different Medicare administrative contractors (MACs) around the country. The MACs receive, review, and pay Medicare claims for health care services provided in their respective regions.

Medicare has undergone many changes over the years. The original Medicare program was designed to pay for hospital stays and physician visits and operated on an indemnity insurance model. In the early 1970s, outpatient physical therapy was added as a covered benefit. Payment models used by Medicare to pay for services have continually evolved since the program's inception. These new payment models have profoundly influenced the physical therapist practice, including documentation.

Part A

Medicare Part A was originally designed to cover inpatient hospital stays. Most patients do not pay a premium to receive Medicare Part A. Part A coverage has been expanded to pay for care provided in post–acute care settings, such as inpatient rehabilitation hospitals, skilled nursing facilities (SNFs), and home health agencies. Medicare uses different payment models in each of these care settings.

Acute Care Hospital Reimbursement

Initially, Medicare Part A paid hospitals using a fee-for-service model of reimbursement. In the 1980s, CMS introduced a prospective payment model in which the hospital receives a lump sum payment based on the patient's diagnosis. Upon discharge, the patient is classified into a diagnosis-related group (DRG) based on his or her diagnosis and severity of illness.[8] The hospital receives a lump sum payment to cover the whole hospital stay (episode) based on the patient's DRG grouping. Payment will not be increased if the care provided costs more than the lump sum payment. The lump sum is often reduced if the patient is discharged quickly to another care setting. The goal of this payment mechanism is for hospitals to provide care as efficiently as possible and reduce the length of hospital stays while encouraging effective discharge planning. Additional incentives have been incorporated into the DRG system to promote value and quality of care. For example, hospitals with high rates of patient complications (like hospital-acquired infections, patient falls, patients readmitted to the hospital within 30 days, etc) may have their DRG payment rates reduced.[8]

Inpatient Rehabilitation Facilities

An inpatient rehabilitation facility (IRF) provides comprehensive rehabilitation to patients after serious illness or injury. An IRF can be a freestanding facility or a unit within an acute care hospital. To qualify for IRF admission, a patient must be able to tolerate a minimum of 3 hours of therapy per day.[9] Upon admission to an IRF, a patient is evaluated by a physician and an interprofessional team of physical, occupational, and speech therapists, rehabilitation nurses, and orthotists/prosthetists.

Medicare reimburses IRFs using a prospective payment system. The IRF receives a lump sum payment that is based on patient characteristics like age, diagnosis, comorbidities, functional status, and cognitive status.[9] Much like the DRG payment system in acute care hospitals, the episode-based payment provides an incentive for the IRF to provide care in an efficient manner. To insure IRFs are admitting the patients most likely to benefit from the services provided by the facilities, Medicare requires that 60% of a facility's caseload be made up of patients with particular diagnoses (eg, stroke, spinal cord injury, brain injury, amputation, etc).[9] An IRF's payment may be reduced for a patient whose stay is interrupted (eg, when a patient is transferred back to the acute care hospital).

In 2014, the Improving Medicare Post-Acute Care Transformation (IMPACT) Act[10] was signed into law. The primary purpose of the IMPACT Act is to standardize the data collected and reported by IRFs and other post–acute care facilities, such as SNFs and home health agencies. Historically, IRFs, SNFs, and home health agencies have used different patient assessment instruments, making comparisons across settings difficult. By gradually standardizing the data collected in these settings, data can be analyzed to determine which care settings can provide the most effective, efficient care for patients based on their health conditions and other characteristics.

For IRFs, new quality reporting requirements have been added, and the requirement that facilities report Functional Independence Measure scores on all patients has been rescinded.[11] Physical therapists working in these facilities must keep abreast of ongoing changes in documentation requirements and payment incentives. Links to setting-specific resources are provided in Table 12-1.

Skilled Nursing Facilities and Subacute Care Units

Some hospitalized patients who are not medically stable enough to go home may not need, or be able to tolerate, the intensity of services offered in an IRF. SNFs are another post–acute care option to prepare patients to return home. SNFs can be freestanding, or they can be units within hospitals or nursing homes. Medicare uses a per day payment model to reimburse SNF care. As of this writing, CMS is transitioning to a new Patient-Driven Payment Model (PDPM) for SNFs.[12] Beginning October 1, 2019, SNFs will receive a daily payment rate based on the needs of the patient (ie, the patient's medical condition, comorbidities, and functional status will determine the daily payment rate). The per diem payment will be adjusted downward the longer the patient stays.

This new model replaces a payment system in place since 1998 that was based on the number of minutes of therapy the patient received per week. Critics of the old system claim it encouraged overutilization because more minutes of therapy were delivered to some patients with the goal of earning higher payments. The new PDPM is designed to reduce incentives for overutilization.[13] As noted previously, new documentation and data collection requirements are likely to emerge as implementation of the IMPACT Act continues. Data will be gathered and analyzed to evaluate how well the system promotes quality of care and overall value compared with other post–acute care settings.

Home Health Care

After discharge from a hospital, rehabilitation facility, or SNF, some patients are still in need of skilled therapy or nursing services. Home health agencies send physical therapists, nurses, and other providers into the patient's home to deliver the necessary care. The patient is assessed using a comprehensive evaluation tool called the Outcome and Assessment Information Set (OASIS).[14] The OASIS tool collects information about the patient's medical condition

TABLE 12-1	
BILLING AND PAYMENT RESOURCES	
GENERAL	http://www.apta.org/Payment http://medpac.gov/-documents-/payment-basics
CODING	http://www.apta.org/Payment/CodingBilling http://www.ama-assn.org/amaone/cpt-current-procedural-terminology http://www.cms.gov/medicare/coding/icd10
MEDICARE ADMINISTRATIVE CONTRACTORS	http://www.cms.gov/Medicare/Medicare-Contracting/Medicare-Administrative-Contractors/MedicareAdministrativeContractors.html
PRIVATE INSURANCE	http://www.apta.org/Payment/PrivateInsurance
OUTPATIENT SETTINGS	http://www.cms.gov/Medicare/Billing/TherapyServices/index.html
INPATIENT REHAB	http://www.cms.gov/Medicare/Medicare-Fee-for-Service-Payment/InpatientRehabFacPPS/index.html
SKILLED NURSING FACILITY	https://www.cms.gov/Medicare/Medicare-Fee-for-Service-Payment/SNFPPS/index.html
LONG-TERM CARE HOSPITALS	http://www.cms.gov/Medicare/Medicare-Fee-for-Service-Payment/LongTermCareHospitalPPS/index.html
HOME HEALTH	http://www.cms.gov/Medicare/Medicare-Fee-for-Service-Payment/HomeHealthPPS/index.html

and functional status. Beginning January 1, 2020, Medicare is implementing a new payment model for home health. The Patient-Driven Grouping Model will pay home health agencies for 30-day episodes of care. Payment amounts will be based on the admission source (ie, whether the patient was recently discharged from the hospital); timing (how long the patient has been receiving home health services); and the patient's diagnosis, functional status (based on the OASIS assessment), and comorbidities.[15]

The PDPM in skilled nursing and the Patient-Driven Grouping Model in home health are examples of an increased payer focus on quality and value of care over volume of care. Physical therapists need to be skilled in documenting accurate and timely assessment of patient function, use of evidence-based interventions, application of clinical practice guidelines, and outcomes of care.

Part B

Medicare Part B pays for care provided by physicians and certain outpatient services, including outpatient physical therapy. Unlike Medicare Part A, patients must pay a monthly premium to receive Medicare Part B. The amount of the premium varies based on income, and it is adjusted

each year.[16] It is possible for a patient to have Medicare Part A but not Medicare Part B if the patient chooses not to pay the Part B premium.

Medicare Part B pays for physical therapy services using a fee-for-service model. Each procedure (or service) provided by the physical therapist is weighted using a system of relative value units (RVUs). The RVU system takes into account the practice expense, work expense, and malpractice/liability expense of each individual procedure.[17] Each procedure's RVU weight is multiplied by a conversion factor and a geographic adjustment that determines how much the therapist will be paid for the procedure.[17] The RVU payment system is used to develop the Medicare Physician Fee Schedule, which is updated annually.[17]

Because paying by individual procedures can lead to overutilization of services, Medicare has implemented several cost-control mechanisms. For example, physical therapy claims are reviewed to make sure the frequency, duration, and content of patient visits are appropriate for the patient's health condition. Other cost-control mechanisms under Medical Part B include claims reviews and audits. Medicare MACs and auditors may request and review physical therapy documentation to make sure it complies with standards outlined in Chapter 15 of the *Medicare Benefit Policy Manual*.[18] The manual states that the physical therapist must develop a plan of care for each patient based on the physical therapy examination. The examination must include standard functional measures such as those described in Chapter 8.[18] The initial plan of care must then be reviewed and certified (signed) by a physician.[18] The plan of care must be recertified by a physician at least once every 90 days or sooner if indicated in the original plan of care.[18] The manual also requires that the physical therapist reassess the patient at least once every 10 visits and report on the patient's progress related to the initial plan of care.[18] If a physical therapist assistant is involved in the patient's care, he or she may document interim treatment notes, but the supervising therapist is responsible for documenting the initial examination and plan of care, subsequent progress reports, and a discharge summary.[18]

Starting January 1, 2019, many physical therapists in outpatient practice have been required to participate in the Merit-based Incentive Payment System (MIPS). The MIPS program requires physical therapists to document information on at least 6 quality measures on at least 60% of their patients.[19] CMS maintains a website for clinicians to find these quality measures (https://qpp.cms.gov/mips/explore-measures/quality-measures). After selecting the year, scroll down and select "Physical Therapy" in the Specialty Measure Set drop-down menu). The MIPS program provides financial incentives for physical therapists to document elements of patient care that are already considered best practice, such as listing the patient's current medications and using functional outcome assessment tools.

The MIPS program will continue to evolve. Additional measures for quality, cost, and improvement activities will likely be added, and payment incentives will be adjusted each year. Physical therapists should expect more Medicare Part B payment reforms in the future. For example, a current proposal from CMS would reduce the payment for services provided by physical therapist assistants starting in 2022.[20] If allowed to go into effect, services provided by physical therapist assistants would be paid at 85% of the fee schedule amount.[20]

Part C

The Balanced Budget Act of 1997 created the option for Medicare recipients to enroll in managed care plans in place of traditional Medicare Parts A and B. Originally called "Medicare+Choice" plans, these managed care products are delivered by private managed care organizations. Now known as "Medicare Advantage," these plans may provide coverage for services not covered under traditional Medicare, such as expanded prescription drug coverage, dental and vision benefits, and health club memberships.[21] Medicare pays the managed care plan a monthly fee, and many Medicare Advantage enrollees also pay a monthly premium.[21] Medicare Advantage plans operate like other managed care plans using a variety of cost-containment methods described earlier in the chapter.

Part D

Part D was added to Medicare in 2006 to provide coverage for prescription drugs. Part D allows Medicare recipients to enroll in private prescription insurance plans or a Medicare Part C plan that offers coverage for prescription drugs.

PROCESSES FOR MANAGING REIMBURSEMENT CLAIMS

As noted earlier in the chapter, Medicare is one of many third-party payers of health care in the United States. However, Medicare often serves as a useful model for learning about reimbursement. Many other insurance companies and plans model their reimbursement policies after Medicare. In some settings, such as skilled nursing and home health, Medicare is the most common payer source.

Regardless of whether the patient has social insurance like Medicare, employer-sponsored insurance, or privately purchased insurance, the process for submitting claims for reimbursement is very similar. The process begins before care is delivered to verify the patient's insurance benefits. After care is provided and documented, information about the encounter is converted into codes that are transmitted to an electronic billing system to the insurance plan for payment. This process is described in more detail in the remainder of the chapter.

Before Care Is Delivered

When a patient is referred to outpatient physical therapy or admitted to an inpatient facility, the patient is registered. Registration involves collecting demographic, contact, and insurance information about the patient. If a patient has previously received care at the same facility, the registration process may simply involve updating the information currently on file. When registering a patient, you should make a photocopy of the patient's insurance card. The back of the card may include important information, so you should copy both sides. If a patient is covered by more than one insurance plan, you should obtain information for all the plans. Any documents that accompany the patient, such as written referrals or copies of relevant documents from other providers, should be collected and placed in the patient's medical record.

Next, the patient's insurance benefits should be verified. If your clinic or practice has a contractual agreement with the patient's insurance company, your billing office should have information for completing this step. If not, use the information from the patient's insurance card to contact

Figure 12-1. Example of an *ICD-10* code.

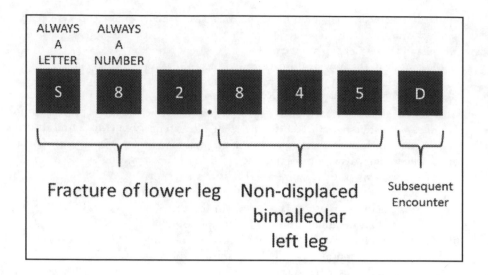

ALWAYS A LETTER   ALWAYS A NUMBER

S 8 2 . 8 4 5 D

Fracture of lower leg   Non-displaced bimalleolar left leg   Subsequent Encounter

the insurance plan for more information. It is important to verify insurance benefits in case the patient's coverage has been canceled or expired. Also, if the patient is covered by more than one insurance plan, you will need to determine which one will be the primary payer.

Besides verifying that the patient has insurance coverage, you also need to find out what information is required for coverage of the services you plan to provide and if there are any services that the insurance company excludes. In many settings, insurance plans will require the provider to submit referrals, examination results, or other documentation in order to preauthorize payment before care is provided.

During Patient Care

After care is initiated, information about the patient and the care provided needs to be documented and converted to a format that can be transmitted to the insurance company. This process is called coding. Both the patient's diagnosis and the treatment provided are typically converted into codes.

Diagnosis Coding

The World Health Organization (who developed the International Classification, Disability and Health model discussed in earlier chapters) also publishes a coding system for diseases, injuries, and other health conditions. This coding system is known as the *International Classification of Diseases, Tenth Revision (ICD-10)*. Information on ordering manuals of the US version of the *ICD-10* is available on the US Centers for Disease Control and Prevention website at http://www.cdc.gov/nchs/icd/icd10.htm. Other publishers sell coding manuals and software specific to different health care professions, including physical therapy. *ICD-10* coding is built into many electronic health records systems (See Chapter 6).

Codes in *ICD-10* include 3 to 7 characters. The first character is always a letter, and the second character is always a number. The first 3 characters provide the main category of the diagnosis with respect to the body region and/or system. The first 3 characters are followed by a period (.). The next 3 characters provide information regarding the specific anatomical site, etiology, and other details. The final seventh character is used for some codes to designate if the patient is being seen for the very first encounter for this condition, if it is a subsequent or follow-up visit, or if the patient is being seen to address sequelae, or a complication, of the diagnosis.

An example of an *ICD-10* code is provided in Figure 12-1. The specifics of *ICD-10* coding are beyond the scope of this text. More information and resources regarding *ICD-10* coding can be found at www.apta.org/ICD10 and www.cms.gov/Medicare/Coding/ICD10/.

Coding for Procedures

In many settings, the Current Procedural Terminology (CPT) coding system is used to describe treatments provided to patients. The American Medical Association publishes and copyrights the CPT code set. Coding manuals can be purchased directly from the American Medical Association or from book retailers. Other publishers offer coding manuals tailored to specific professions or care settings.

CPT codes consist of 5 numeric digits. For example, CPT codes 97161, 97162, and 92163 are used to indicate that a physical therapy evaluation was performed.[22] Table 12-2 lists many of the codes physical therapists use frequently. Many of the codes stipulate that the provider must provide direct one-on-one contact with the patient throughout the treatment period. Many codes are "timed" codes that specify treatment should be provided in 15-minute increments. According to the CPT coding manual, a 15-minute "unit" can be billed when at least half of the 15-minute time has

TABLE 12-2

CURRENT PROCEDURAL TERMINOLOGY CODES COMMONLY USED BY PHYSICAL THERAPISTS

Author's note: This brief list is a sample of CPT codes that may be used by physical therapists. For a more comprehensive listing, please consult a CPT coding manual available from the American Medical Association. Individual payers may reimburse some codes but not others. You should check with the payer to determine coverage.

CODE	DESCRIPTION	TIMED CODE?
97161	Physical Therapist Evaluation—Low Complexity	No
97162	Physical Therapist Evaluation—Moderate Complexity	No
97163	Physical Therapist Evaluation—High Complexity	No
97164	Physical Therapy Re-evaluation	No

Unattended Therapeutic Modalities

Author's note: For those modalities, the physical therapist (or physical therapist assistant under the physical therapist's supervision) sets up the modality, provides patient instruction, and provides ongoing supervision during the treatment.

CODE	DESCRIPTION	TIMED CODE?
97010	Hot packs/cold packs	No
97012	Mechanical traction	No
97014	Electrical stimulation	No
97016	Vasopneumatic devices	No
97018	Paraffin bath	No
97022	Whirlpool	No
97024	Diathermy	No

Constant Attendance Therapeutic Modalities

Author's note: For these modalities, the physical therapist (or physical therapist assistant under the physical therapist's supervision) sets up the modality and provides patient instruction. The physical therapist (or physical therapist assistant) must provide direct, one-on-one patient contact throughout the procedure.; these codes are timed in 15-minute increments.

CODE	DESCRIPTION	TIMED CODE?
97032	Electrical stimulation	Yes
97033	Iontophoresis	Yes
97034	Contrast baths	Yes
97035	Ultrasound	Yes
97036	Hubbard tank	Yes *(continued)*

elapsed.[17] If the treatment lasts more than 15 minutes, additional units can be billed once the halfway point of the next unit has been passed.[23] The following are examples of this:

- 1 unit = at least 8 minutes of treatment
- 2 units = at least 23 minutes of treatment provided
- 3 units = at least 38 minutes of treatment provided
- 4 units = at least 53 minutes of treatment provided

Sometimes, a CPT code alone does not adequately describe the services provided to this patient. In these cases, modifiers should be added. Modifiers are 2-character codes that can include both numbers and letters. For example, the modifier -GP added to any CPT code indicates that the service was performed by a physical therapist. Another common example is modifier -59.[23] There are therapeutic procedures that are similar and may overlap with each

	TABLE 12-2 (CONTINUED)	
	CURRENT PROCEDURAL TERMINOLOGY CODES COMMONLY USED BY PHYSICAL THERAPISTS	

Therapeutic Procedures

Author's note: For all except 97150, the physical therapist (or physical therapist assistant) must provide direct, one-on-one patient contact throughout the procedure; codes are timed in 15-minute increments. Code 97150 is untimed and can only be billed once per visit.

97110	Therapeutic exercise (strength, endurance, flexibility)	Yes
97112	Neuromuscular reeducation (movement, balance, coordination, proprioception)	Yes
CODE	**DESCRIPTION**	**TIMED CODE?**
97113	Aquatic therapy	Yes
97116	Gait training	Yes
97124	Massage	Yes
97140	Manual therapy techniques	Yes
97150	Group, 2 or more individuals	No
97530	Therapeutic activities	Yes
97533	Sensory integration	Yes
97535	Self-care/Home management	Yes

Reprinted with permission from the American Medical Association. 2012.

other. Aquatic therapy involves exercise in the water. If a physical therapist performed aquatic exercises with a patient, it would be inappropriate to bill both CPT codes 97110 (therapeutic exercise) and 97113 (aquatic therapy) for that treatment.[23] However, if a therapist instructs a patient in land-based exercises for 15 minutes and then spends another 15 minutes on aquatic exercise, it would be appropriate to code and bill for both of these procedures. The therapist would add the -59 modifier to indicate that the 2 procedures were provided to the patient at distinctly different times.

As you document patient care, keep in mind that documentation in the medical record will often be compared with the codes (both diagnostic and procedure codes) listed on the insurance claim. Your documentation must support the *ICD-10* and CPT codes listed on the claim. For example, there are 3 codes that can be used to bill for a physical therapy examination. One of the 3 codes is used to designate the level of complexity of the patient's condition and the therapist's clinical decision making. In order to use the code for a "high-complexity" physical therapy evaluation (97163), the therapist must document the following[22]:

- The patient has 3 or more comorbidities or other personal factors that will impact their recovery.

- The examination identified the need for intervention addressing 4 or more impairments, activity limitations, and/or participation restrictions.
- The patient's clinical condition is currently unstable.
- The patient's overall condition requires a high level of clinical decision making to outline a safe, effective plan of care.

If one or more of these elements is not accurately documented, the use of the code for a "high-complexity" physical therapy evaluation would not be supported. The evaluation would need to be coded as either "moderate" or "low" complexity (97161 or 97162) based on the documentation. Careful, thorough documentation is essential to support which of the 3 codes is used.

Billing

Once data regarding the patient and the care provided to the patient are translated into codes, these codes are entered into an electronic billing system. These forms are then submitted to the insurance company (or regional MAC in the case of Medicare) for payment. Traditionally, bills were printed on paper and submitted to the insurer via postal mail. Now, bills are generating and transmitted to insurers electronically. This means most health care facilities use health information technology not just to document patient care but also to run most aspects of their business. More on health informatics and electronic health records is available in Chapter 6.

Claims Denials and Appeals

After you submit a health insurance claim, the insurer reviews and processes the claim. If there are problems with the claim, the insurer may deny payment. The insurer typically sends a notice of the denial, called an Explanation of Benefits to the patient and the provider. If the claim was denied for technical errors (such as missing information on the claim form, minor coding problems, etc), the provider can fix the problems and resubmit the claim. If the claim was denied for a coverage issue (eg, the documentation does not demonstrate medical necessity or provision of skilled service or the treatment provided or health condition is excluded by the insurance plan), the payer and/or patient may file an appeal.

You should appeal a claim denial if you believe the care you provided met the coverage requirements of the insurance plan and that the documentation proves you provided reasonable, necessary skilled care. Medicare's appeal process is outlined on the CMS website.[24] Managed care, employer-based, and private health plans should also have appeals processes. You can often find these on the insurance company's website, in the provider contract agreement, or by contacting the insurer directly.

Appealing a claim denial takes time, meaning you may not get paid for services provided for several months. Appeals also require time and attention from the clinician and billing staff. Therefore, it is always better to prevent a denial than to file an appeal. Some strategies for preventing denials are as follows:

- **Make sure your documentation and billing are accurate and consistent.** It is not uncommon for payers to request copies of your documentation for review. Your documentation must be complete and support the treatment provided. Never change your documentation after it is complete. Although it may be tempting to go back and add details later, if you change a note after copies are already shared with insurers or others, it could be perceived as fraud. (Please see Chapter 3 for more on fraud, waste, and abuse.)
- **Carefully read and understand the CPT code descriptions.** CPT coding manuals provide descriptors to help determine which code is the best to use for a specific procedure or service. For example, CPT codes 97110 and 97112 are both listed as "therapeutic procedures."[23] The description for code 97110 clarifies that this code should be used for therapeutic exercises to improve strength, endurance, range of motion, or flexibility.[23] The description for code 97112 states this code should be used for exercises related to balance, coordination, and proprioception.[23] Also, when using timed CPT

codes, make sure the treatment times listed for each procedure and the total treatment time are accurate. When documenting, some clinicians will refer to the actual CPT code in their documentation. Regardless, you should strive to use language that demonstrates skilled services were performed and the services match the descriptions of the CPT codes billed.

- **Be aware of insurance exclusions and limitations.** If you provide a treatment to a patient that you feel the insurer will not cover, you should discuss this with your patient before providing the service so the patient has an opportunity to give informed consent (see Chapter 3). In some cases, if the patient chooses to receive the treatment after being notified that insurance will not pay for it, the patient may be billed directly for the service. Medicare requires the use of an advance beneficiary notice to document the patient's consent.[25,26]
- **Make documentation understandable for both professionals and the lay public.** To be understandable, documentation must be legible. If you write notes by hand, your penmanship must be easy to read. Illegible notes frustrate readers who may not be able to decipher important information that supports the insurance claim. Illegible notes can also lead to medical errors and jeopardize patient safety. With the wide implementation of electronic health records (See Chapter 13), handwritten notes are becoming much less common.

    Another important way to make documentation understandable is to limit abbreviations and avoid jargon. Even if a fellow therapist can read and understand your notes, other readers who do not have the same professional training may not be familiar with the terminology and abbreviations we use every day. This makes it hard for readers to follow your decision-making process and to determine whether the patient received necessary skilled care. Use only standard abbreviations, and write your documentation with the layperson in mind.
- **Show skill and integrate CPT code terminology when describing interventions in the Objective section and plan of care.** General descriptions of interventions that do not include the parameters of treatment do not demonstrate skilled care. Remember to describe how your involvement was necessary. Also, consider using CPT code language in our descriptions. For example, use the words "gait training" instead of "ambulation." Then, describe the things you did during that intervention that were skilled. Did you advance or make adjustments to the parameters of the treatment or activity? Did you provide instruction or correction? Did you provide skillful, hands-on facilitation, support, or inhibition of movement? Make it clear to all readers why a licensed physical therapist was required to provide the intervention.

- **Cultivate good documentation habits.** The life of a physical therapist is hectic, and creating quality documentation can be time consuming. Unfortunately, some clinicians take "shortcuts" when documenting that may seem efficient at the time but can lead to claims denials later. Taking shortcuts can lead to inaccurate documents or documents that fail to demonstrate the need for services, provision of skilled care, or patient progress.

  Documentation is most accurate when it is completed during or immediately following care delivery. You may forget important details if hours (or days) pass between care delivery and documentation. Although not every note can be completed during the treatment session, you should always complete documentation the same day care was delivered. Besides inviting claims denials, incomplete and inaccurate notes can present patient safety and legal liability risks (see Chapter 3 for a discussion of fraud, waste, and abuse).

  Be careful to avoid using phrases that tell the reader nothing. For example, writing "Tolerated treatment well" in the Assessment does not provide any information about how the patient actually tolerated treatment. Did the patient report less pain or fatigue? Was the patient able to tolerate more exercises or activity? Did the patient ask questions, and how did you answer these questions? Paint a picture for the reader to illustrate the patient's response to treatment and any progress made so your decision-making process is clear.

  Similarly, avoid writing phrases like "Continue as above" or "Follow" in the Plan portion of the note. Readers will look to the plan of care to find out how you are progressing the patient's treatment over time. The use of these phrases does not show progress. Instead, clearly document the interventions provided in the Objective section (see Chapter 8), and in the Plan, tell the reader what you will be doing with the patient at the next visit.

- **Engage in peer chart review audits to improve quality of documentation and patient care.** In many practices, physical therapists provide peer audits of medical records to develop and improve documentation quality. The American Physical Therapy Association recommends that peer reviews of physical therapy services should be completed by physical therapists.[27] Peer reviews may focus, for example, on the specific contents of each section of the documentation, how well the documentation demonstrates medical necessity and skilled care, and how well the documentation in the medical record supports the codes used to bill for services provided. The American Physical Therapy Association's Defensible Documentation website (http://www.apta.org/DefensibleDocumentation) provides sample checklists that can be used as starting points to develop audit tools for your practice.

SUMMARY

Documentation by the physical therapist is an integral component of the billing and payment process. Documentation requirements and practices continue to evolve due to developments in technology, changes in the US health care system, and efforts to reduce fraud, waste, and abuse. As payers (and society) demand more value for their health care dollar, physical therapists must be accountable for producing complete, accurate, and defensible documentation that supports billing claims.

REVIEW QUESTIONS

1. How does insurance protect patients from financial risk? How might this protection impact patients' choices regarding their health care? How might this protection impact the behavior of health care providers?

2. What is the difference between a premium and a copayment? How might these mechanisms impact patient behavior with respect to seeking health care?

3. What is meant by the term managed care?

4. How does Medicare pay for care delivered in acute care hospitals? Inpatient rehab facilities? Skilled nursing facilities? Home health agencies? Outpatient physical therapy clinics?

5. What is the difference between *ICD-10* codes and CPT codes?

6. What steps can you take to reduce the risk that insurance claims will be denied?

APPLICATION EXERCISES

1. Review an interim/daily note for an outpatient (it could be a patient either you or a colleague treated). From the description of the interventions provided, determine which CPT codes should be used on the reimbursement claim form.

2. Review an initial examination note written by a classmate, clinical instructor, or colleague. Critique the note from an insurance company's perspective. Share your feedback with the author of the note.

3. In the clinic, choose a patient whose care you documented. Working with the clinic staff, follow the reimbursement claim from filing to final payment. During the process, take note of how many people had access to the medical record. Was payment obtained on the first attempt? How could documentation be improved?

4. For each of the following scenarios, what CPT code(s) would be used to bill for the services provided? Include quantity for each CPT code. How would you describe

each intervention in your documentation to demonstrate skilled services were provided?

   a. Documentation indicates Mrs. J received 14 minutes of manual therapy and 16 minutes of flexibility and strengthening exercises.

   b. Mr. J received 12 minutes of gait training followed by 10 minutes of exercises for balance and proprioception.

   c. Sam D. received 10 minutes of warm whirlpool to the left ankle and foot, 10 minutes of exercises for ankle flexibility and range of motion, and 10 minutes of exercises for balance and proprioception.

REFERENCES

1. Kaiser Family Foundation. Health insurance coverage of the total population 2017. State Health Facts website. https://www.kff.org/other/state-indicator/total-population/?currentTimeframe=0&sortModel=%7B%22colId%22:%22Location%22,%22sort%22:%22asc%22%7D. Accessed April 5, 2019.

2. Goddeeris JH. Payment reform and "bending the curve." In: Meyer DJ, ed. *Economics of Health*. Kalamazoo, MI: W.E. Upjohn Institute for Employment Research; 2016:51-80.

3. Abrams MK, Nuzum R, Zezza MA, Ryan J, Kiszla J, Guterman S. Affordable Care Act's payment and delivery system reforms: a progress report at five years. The Commonwealth Fund website. https://www.commonwealthfund.org/publications/issue-briefs/2015/may/affordable-care-acts-payment-and-delivery-system-reforms. Updated May 7, 2015. Accessed April 5, 2019.

4. Centers for Medicare & Mediciaid Services. Accountable Care Organizations (ACOs): general information. CMS Innovation Center website. https://innovation.cms.gov/initiatives/aco/. Updated April 11, 2019. Accessed April 14, 2019.

5. Medicare Payment Advisory Commission. Accountable Care Organization payment systems. MedPAC Payment Basics website. http://medpac.gov/docs/default-source/payment-basics/medpac_payment_basics_18_aco_final_sec.pdf?sfvrsn=0. Updated October 2018. Accessed April 5, 2019.

6. Centers for Medicare & Mediciaid Services. What's Medicare? Medicare.gov website. https://www.medicare.gov/what-medicare-covers/your-medicare-coverage-choices/whats-medicare. Accessed April 5, 2019.

7. Centers for Medicare & Mediciaid Services. Program history. Medicaid.gov website. https://www.medicaid.gov/about-us/program-history/index.html. Accessed April 5, 2019.

8. Medicare Payment Advisory Commission. Hospital acute inpatient services payment system. MedPAC Payment Basics website. http://medpac.gov/docs/default-source/payment-basics/medpac_payment_basics_18_hospital_final_v2_sec.pdf?sfvrsn=0. Updated October 2018. Accessed April 5, 2019.

9. Medicare Payment Advisory Commission. Inpatient rehabilitation facilities payment system. MedPAC Payment Basics website. http://medpac.gov/docs/default-source/payment-basics/medpac_payment_basics_18_irf_final_sec.pdf?sfvrsn=0. Updated October 2018. Accessed April 5, 2019.

10. Centers for Medicare & Mediciaid Services. IMPACT Act of 2014 data standardization & cross setting measures. Post-Acute Quality Initiatives website. https://www.cms.gov/Medicare/Quality-Initiatives-Patient-Assessment-Instruments/Post-Acute-Care-Quality-Initiatives/IMPACT-Act-of-2014/IMPACT-Act-of-2014-Data-Standardization-and-Cross-Setting-Measures.html. Updated December 11, 2018. Accessed April 5, 2019.

11. Centers for Medicare & Mediciaid Services. Fiscal year 2019 Medicare inpatient rehabilitation facility prospective payment system final rule (CMS-688-F). CMS.gov Newsroom website. https://www.cms.gov/newsroom/fact-sheets/fiscal-year-2019-medicare-inpatient-rehabilitation-facility-prospective-payment-system-final-rule. Updated July 31, 2018. Accessed April 5, 2019.

12. Centers for Medicare & Mediciaid Services. Patient driven payment model. Skilled Nursing Facility PPS website. https://www.cms.gov/Medicare/Medicare-Fee-for-Service-Payment/SNFPPS/PDPM.html. Accessed April 14, 2019.

13. American Physical Therapy Association. Fact sheet: 2019 skilled nursing facility prospective payment system final rule. Medicare Payment and Policies for Skilled Nursing Facilities website. http://www.apta.org/Payment/Medicare/CodingBilling/SNF/FactSheet/2018/8/9/. Updated August 9, 2018. Accessed April 5, 2019.

14. Medicare Payment Advisory Commission. Home health care services payment system. MedPAC Payment Basics website. http://medpac.gov/docs/default-source/payment-basics/medpac_payment_basics_18_hha_final_sec.pdf?sfvrsn=0. Updated October 2018. Accessed April 5, 2019.

15. Centers for Medicare & Mediciaid Services. Home health patient-driven groupings model - split implementation. Medicare Learning Network website. https://www.cms.gov/Outreach-and-Education/Medicare-Learning-Network-MLN/MLNMattersArticles/Downloads/MM11081.pdf. Updated February 15, 2019. Accessed April 5, 2019.

16. Centers for Medicare & Mediciaid Services. Part B costs. Your Medicare Costs website. https://www.medicare.gov/your-medicare-costs/part-b-costs. Accessed April 15, 2019.

17. Medicare Payment Advisory Commission. Outpatient therapy services payment system. MedPAC Payment Basics website. http://medpac.gov/docs/default-source/payment-basics/medpac_payment_basics_18_opt_final_sec.pdf?sfvrsn=0. Updated October 2018. Accessed April 11, 2019.

18. Centers for Medicare & Mediciaid Services. Chapter 15 - covered medical and other health services. *Medicare Benefit Policy Manual* website. https://www.cms.gov/Regulations-and-Guidance/Guidance/Manuals/downloads/bp102c15.pdf. Updated February 1, 2019. Accessed April 11, 2019.

19. Smith H. MIPS is here: this is what you need to know. *PT in Motion*. 2019;11(3):10-13.

20. American Physical Therapy Association. A permanent fix to the therapy cap: improved access for Medicare patients comes with a pending APTA-opposed cut to PTA payment. *PT in Motion* News website. http://www.apta.org/PTinMotion/News/2018/02/09/TherapyCapRepeal/. Updated February 9, 2018. Accessed April 4, 2019.

21. Medicare Payment Advisory Commission. Medicare Advantage program payment system. MedPAC Payment Basics website. http://medpac.gov/docs/default-source/payment-basics/medpac_payment_basics_18_ma_final_sec.pdf?sfvrsn=0. Updated October 2018. Accessed April 11, 2019.

22. Evans WK. Compliance matters: documenting the new evaluation codes. *PT in Motion*. 2017;9(2):8-13.

23. Fearon HM, Cohn R, Rausch RW. *Coding and Payment Guide for the Physical Therapist 2016*. West Valley City, UT: Optum360; 2015.

24. Centers for Medicare & Mediciaid Services. Medicare Parts A and B appeals process. Medicare Learning Network website. https://www.cms.gov/Outreach-and-Education/Medicare-Learning-Network-xLN/MLNProducts/downloads/medicareappealsprocess.pdf. Updated October 2018. Accessed April 11, 2019.

25. Centers for Medicare & Mediciaid Services. Medicare advanced written notices of noncoverage. Medicare Learning Network website. https://www.cms.gov/Outreach-and-Education/Medicare-Learning-Network-MLN/MLNProducts/downloads/abn_booklet_icn006266.pdf. Updated October 2018. Accessed April 11, 2019.

26. Centers for Medicare & Mediciaid Services. Outpatient therapy services and advanced beneficiary notice of noncoverage, Form CMS-R-131. Therapy Services website. https://www.cms.gov/Medicare/Billing/TherapyServices/Downloads/2018-08-ABN-FAQ.pdf. Updated August 2018. Accessed April 11, 2019.

27. American Physical Therapy Association. Peer review resources. APTA website. http://www.apta.org/PeerReview/. Update March 2016. Accessed July 6, 2019.

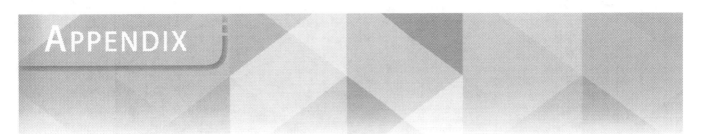

Abbreviations and Symbols

This list provides many of the abbreviations and symbols used in medical charts and in physical therapy records. Because documentation styles can vary, you should check with your facility regarding abbreviations and symbols that are "approved" for use. Also, note that some abbreviations have more than one meaning. Be careful and understand the context in which each abbreviation is used.

ABBREVIATIONS

A

(A), (a), @, or ⓐ	assist	AE	above elbow
A: or A	assessment	AFB	acid-fast bacilli
AAROM	active assistive range of motion	AFO	ankle-foot orthosis
Ab	antibody	AGA	appropriate for gestational age
abd	abduction	AIDS	acquired immunodeficiency syndrome
ABG(s)	arterial blood gas(es)		
ABN	advanced beneficiary notice	AK	above knee
ac	before meals	AKA	above knee amputation
ACE	angiotensin-converting enzyme	ALL	acute lymphoblastic leukemia
Ach	acetylcholine	ALS	amyotrophic lateral sclerosis
ACL	anterior cruciate ligament	am	before noon
ACO	accountable care organization	AMA	against medical advice; American Medical Association
AD	assistive device; Alzheimer's disease		
ADA	Americans with Disabilities Act	AMB	ambulatory; ambulate; ambulation
add	adduction	AML	acute myeloblastic leukemia
ADL	activities of daily living	AMP	Amputee Mobility Predictor
ad lib	as desired	ANOVA	analysis of variance
ADM	abductor digiti minimi	AP	ankle pump; anteroposterior

Erickson ML, Utzman RR, McKnight RS.
Physical Therapy Documentation: From Examination to Outcome,
Third Edition (pp 131-138).
© 2020 Taylor & Francis Group.

APB	abductor pollicis brevis	ARRA	American Recovery and Reinvestment Act
APL	abductor pollicis longus		
APTA	American Physical Therapy Association	ASA	aspirin
		ASAP	as soon as possible
ARDS	adult (acute) respiratory distress syndrome	ASHD	arteriosclerotic heart disease
		ATF	anterior talofibular
AROM	active range of motion	AV	arteriovenous

B

Ba	barium	BMD	bone mineral density
BBB	blood-brain barrier	BMI	body mass index
BE	below elbow	BP	blood pressure
BI	brain injury	BPH	benign prostatic hyperplasia
bid	twice daily	BPM or bpm	beats per minute
BK	below knee	BRP	bathroom privileges
BKA	below knee amputation	BSA	body surface area
BLE or (B)LE	bilateral lower extremities	BUE or (B)UE	bilateral upper extremities
BM	bowel movement	BUN	blood urea nitrogen

C

Ca	calcium	CNS	central nervous system
CA	cancer	c/o or C/O	complains of
CABG	coronary artery bypass graft	COPD	chronic obstructive pulmonary disease
CAD	coronary artery disease		
CAT	computerized axial tomography	CORF	comprehensive outpatient rehabilitation facility
CBC	complete blood count		
c/c or C/C	chief complaint; current condition	COTA	Certified Occupational Therapy Assistant
cc or cm³	cubic centimeter		
CCU	critical (or coronary) care unit	CP	cerebral palsy
CDC	Centers for Disease Control and Prevention	CPAP	continuous positive airway pressure
		CPM	continuous passive motion
C. diff	Clostridium difficile	CPR	cardiopulmonary resuscitation
CDO	care delivery organization	CPT	Current Procedural Terminology
CF	calcaneofibular; cystic fibrosis	CRNP	Certified Registered Nurse Practitioner
CGA	contact guard assist		
CHI	closed head injury	C & S	culture and sensitivity
CHO	carbohydrate	CSF	cerebrospinal fluid
Cl	chlorine	CT	computed tomography
cm	centimeter	CV	cardiovascular
CMC	carpometacarpal	CVA	cerebrovascular accident
CMS	Centers for Medicare & Medicaid Services	CWP	cold whirlpool
		cx	cancel; crutches
CMV	cytomegalovirus		

D

DASH	Disabilities of the Arm, Shoulder, and Hand (outcomes measure)	DD	developmental delay
		DDD	degenerative disc disease
DBS	deep brain stimulator (stimulation)	dep.	dependent
d/c	discharge; discontinue	dept.	department
DC	Doctor of Chiropractic; Chiropractor	DF	dorsiflexion

DHHR	Department of Health and Human Resources	DNR	do not resuscitate
DI	dorsal interossei	DO	Doctor of Osteopathic Medicine
DIP	distal interphalangeal	DOI	date of injury
DJD	degenerative joint disease	DRG	diagnosis-related group
DM	diabetes mellitus	DRUJ	distal radioulnar joint
DME	durable medical equipment	DTR	deep tendon reflex
DMERC	durable medical equipment regional carrier	DVT	deep vein thrombosis
		dx	diagnosis

E

ea.	each	EMS	emergency medical services
EBP	evidence-based practice	ENG	electronystagmograph
ECF	extracellular fluid	EO	elbow orthosis
E. coli	Escherichia coli	EOB	explanation of benefits
ECRB	extensor carpi radialis brevis	EPB	extensor pollicis brevis
ECRL	extensor carpi radialis longus	EPL	extensor pollicis longus
ECU	extensor carpi ulnaris	ER	external rotation; emergency room
ED	emergency department	ERV	expiratory reserve volume
EDC	extensor digitorum communis	ES	effect size; electrical stimulation
EDM	extensor digiti minimi	ESR	erythrocyte sedimentation rate
EEG	electroencephalogram	ESRD	end-stage renal disease
EENT	eyes, ears, nose, and throat	ET	endotracheal
EHR	electronic health record	EtOH or ETOH	ethyl alcohol
EIP	extensor indicis proprius	ev or ever	eversion
EKG, ECG	electrocardiogram	eval.	evaluation
EMG	electromyogram	ex.	exercise
EMR	electronic medical record	EXT	extension

F

F or 3/5	fair (manual muscle test)	FM or FMS	fibromyalgia syndrome
FBS	fasting blood sugar	FO	foot orthosis
FCE	functional capacity evaluation	FOR	functional outcome report
FCR	flexor carpi radialis	FPB	flexor pollicis brevis
FCU	flexor carpi ulnaris	FPL	flexor pollicis longus
FDA	US Food and Drug Administration	FRC	functional residual capacity
FDM	flexor digiti minimi	FSBPT	Federation of State Boards of Physical Therapy
FDP	flexor digitorum profundus		
FDS	flexor digitorum superficialis	FTSG	full-thickness skin graft
FES	functional electrical stimulation	FU or F/U	follow-up
FEV	forced expiratory volume	FUO	fever of unknown origin
FHR	fetal heart rate	FVC	forced vital capacity
FIM	Functional Independence Measure	FWB	full weight bearing
fl	fluid	FWW	front-wheeled walker
FLEX	flexion	fx	fracture

G

G or 4/5	good (manual muscle test)	GH	glenohumeral
g	gram	GI	gastrointestinal
GA	gestational age	GS	gluteal sets
GERD	gastroesophageal reflux disease	GTT	glucose tolerance test

H

H$_2$O	water	HIT	health information technology
h, hr, or hr.	hour	HITECH	Health Information Technology for Economic and Clinical Health Act
HAV	hepatitis A virus; hallux abductovalgus	HIV	human immunodeficiency virus
Hb	hemoglobin	HMO	health maintenance organization
HBV	hepatitis B virus	HNP	herniated nucleus pulposus
HCFA	Health Care Financing Administration	h/o	history of
		HO	hand orthosis; hip orthosis
HCPCS	Healthcare Common Procedure Coding System	HOB	head of bed
		H & P	history and physical
Hct	hematocrit	HP	hot pack
HCV	hepatitis C virus	HPI	history of present illness
HDL	high-density lipoprotein	HR	handrail; heart rate
HEP	home exercise program	HRT	hormone replacement therapy
H & H	hemoglobin and hematocrit	hs	at bedtime
HHA	home health agency	HTN	hypertension
HIPAA	Health Insurance Portability and Accountability Act	hx	history
		Hz	hertz

I

I or (I)	independent	Ig	immunoglobulin
IADL	instrumental activities of daily living	IM	intramuscular
IC	inspiratory capacity	Imp:	overall impression
ICD	*International Classification of Diseases*	IMPACT	Improving Medicare Post-Acute Care Transformation Act
ICF	intracellular fluid; International Classification of Functioning, Disability and Health	INH	isoniazid
		inv	inversion
		I & O	intake and output
ICHI	International Classification of Health Interventions	IP	inpatient; interphalangeal
		IPPS	inpatient prospective payment system
ICP	intracranial pressure		
ICU	intensive care unit	IR	internal rotation
I & D	incision and drainage	IRF	Inpatient Rehabilitation Facility
IDDM	insulin-dependent diabetes mellitus	IRFPAI	Inpatient Rehabilitation Facility Patient Assessment Instrument
IDEA	Individuals with Disabilities Education Act		
		IRV	inspiratory reserve volume
IEP	Individualized Education Plan	IV	intravenous
IFSP	Individualized Family Service Plan		

K

K	potassium	kg	kilogram
KAFO	knee-ankle-foot orthosis	KO	knee orthosis

L

Ⓛ, L, or (L)	left	LDL	low-density lipoprotein
L	liter	LE	lower extremity
LAC	long-arm cast	LHD	left hand dominant
LAQ	long-arc quadriceps exercise	LLC	long leg cast
LCL	lateral collateral ligament	LMN	lower motor neuron

LMRP	local medical review policies	LTFG	long-term functional goal
LP	lumbar puncture	LTG	long-term goal
L/S, l/s	lifestyle	LTM	long-term memory
LT	lunotriquetral		

M

m	meter	MID	multi-infarct dementia
m.	muscle	min	minimal
MAC	Medicare Administrative Contractor	MIPS	Merit-based Incentive Payment System
max	maximum		
MCID	minimal clinically important difference	mm	millimeter
		mm Hg	millimeters of mercury
MCL	medial collateral ligament	MMT	manual muscle test
MCP	metacarpophalangeal	mod	moderate
MD	muscular dystrophy; medical doctor/ physician	MOI	mechanism of injury
		mos	months
MDC	minimal detectable change	MRI	magnetic resonance image
MDS	minimum data set	MRSA	methicillin-resistant *Staphylococcus aureus*
MEDS or meds	medicines, medications		
MG	myasthenia gravis	MTP	metatarsophalangeal
MHz	megahertz	mV	millivolt
MI	myocardial infarction	μV	microvolt

N

N or 5/5	normal (manual muscle test)	NIDDM	noninsulin-dependent diabetes mellitus
N	newton		
n.	nerve	NIH	National Institutes of Health
Na	sodium	NMES	neuromuscular electrical stimulation
N/A	not applicable	NPO	nothing by mouth
NBQC	narrow base quad cane	NSAID(s)	nonsteroidal anti-inflammatory drug(s)
NDI	Neck Disability Index		
NDT	neurodevelopmental treatment	NT	not tested
NICU	neonatal intensive care unit	n & v	nausea and vomiting
		NWB	nonweight bearing

O

O: or O	objective	OP	opponens pollicis; outpatient
O$_2$ or O$_2$	oxygen	OR	operating room
OA	osteoarthritis	ORIF	open reduction internal fixation
OASIS	outcome and assessment information set	OSHA	Occupational Safety & Health Administration
OB/GYN	obstetrics and gynecology	OT	Occupational Therapist
OBS	organic brain syndrome	OTC	over-the-counter (ie, drugs)
OCD	obsessive compulsive disorder	OTR/L	Occupational Therapist Registered and Licensed
ODM	opponens digiti minimi		
OI	osteogenesis imperfecta	oz or oz.	ounce
OOB	out of bed		

P

P or 2/5	poor (manual muscle test)
P: or P	plan
p!	pain
PA	posteroanterior
PA-C	Physician Assistant-Certified
pc	after meals
PCA	patient-controlled anesthesia
PCL	posterior cruciate ligament
PD	Parkinson's disease
PDPM	Patient-Driven Payment Model
PDR	Physicians' Desk Reference
PE	pulmonary embolism
PEG	percutaneous endoscopic gastrostomy (tube)
PERRLA	pupils equal, round (regular), reactive to light, and accommodating
PET	positron emission tomography
PF	plantarflexion
PFT	pulmonary function test
PHI	protected health information
PI	palmar interossei
PIP	proximal interphalangeal
PL	palmaris longus
PLOF	prior level of function
pm	after noon
PMH	past (prior, previous) medical history
PNF	proprioceptive neuromuscular facilitation
PNS	peripheral nervous system
po	by mouth
POMR	problem-oriented medical record
post-op	postoperative
PPO	preferred provider organization
PPACA	Patient Protection and Affordable Care Act
PPS	prospective payment system
PQ	pronator quadratus
Pr:	problem
PRN	as needed
PROM	passive range of motion
PRUJ	proximal radioulnar joint
PT	Physical Therapist; pronator teres; prothrombin time
Pt. or pt.	patient
PTA	Physical Therapist Assistant; prior to admission
PTCA	percutaneous transluminal coronary angioplasty
PTF	posterior talofibular
PTT	partial thromboplastin time
PVD	peripheral vascular disease
PWB	partial weight bearing (usually 50% unless otherwise indicated; may need to check with physician to clarify)

Q

QS or qs	quad set/quadriceps set

R

® or (R)	right
RA	rheumatoid arthritis
RBC	red blood cell
RC	radiocarpal
RCL	radial collateral ligament
RD	radial deviation
RDS	respiratory distress syndrome
reps	repetitions
RGO	reciprocating gait orthosis
RHD	right hand dominant
R/O or r/o	rule out
ROM	range of motion
RPE	rate of perceived exertion
RR	respiratory rate
R/S or r/s	reschedule
RT	respiratory therapy
RTC	return to clinic
RTW	return to work
RUG	resource utilization group
RV	residual volume
RVU	relative value units
Rx	prescription

S

S: or S	subjective
SAC	short-arm cast
SaO_2	oxygen saturation
SAQ	short-arc quadriceps exercise
SBA	stand by assist
SCI	spinal cord injury
SEM	standard error of the measurement
SEWHFO	shoulder-elbow-wrist-hand-finger orthosis
SF-36	Short-Form Health Survey
SIDS	sudden infant death syndrome
SL	scapholunate; side lying
SLC	short leg cast
SLE	systemic lupus erythematosus
SLP	speech language pathologist
SLR	straight leg raise
SMA	spinal muscular atrophy
SNF	skilled nursing facility
SO	shoulder orthosis
SOAP	Subjective, Objective, Assessment, and Plan
SOB	shortness of breath
s/p	status post
SPT	Student Physical Therapist
SPTA	Student Physical Therapist Assistant
s/s	signs and symptoms
ST	scapulothoracic
stat	immediately
STG	short-term goal
STM	short-term memory
STSG	split-thickness skin graft
SVN or s	supervision

T

T or 1/5	trace (manual muscle test)
T	temperature
TA	therapeutic activity
TB	tuberculosis
TBI	traumatic brain injury
T or tbsp	tablespoon
TDWB	touch-down weight bearing
TENS	transcutaneous electrical nerve stimulation
TFCC	triangular fibrocartilaginous complex
THA	total hip arthroplasty
THR	total hip replacement
TIA	transient ischemic attack
tid	three times a day
TJC	The Joint Commission
TKA	total knee arthroplasty
TKE	terminal knee extension
TKR	total knee replacement
TMJ	temporomandibular joint
TP	therapeutic procedure
TPN	total parenteral nutrition
t or tsp	teaspoon
TTP	tender to palpation
TTWB	toe touch weight bearing
TUG	Timed Up and Go
TV	tidal volume
Tx: or tx	traction or treatment

U

UCL	ulnar collateral ligament
UD	ulnar deviation
UE	upper extremity
UMN	upper motor neuron
US	ultrasound
UTI	urinary tract infection
UV	ultraviolet

V

V	volt

W

W	watt
WBAT	weight bearing as tolerated
WBC	white blood cell
WBQC	wide base quad cane
w/c	wheelchair
w/cm² or W/cm²	watts per centimeters squared
WFL	within functional limits
WHFO	wrist-hand-finger orthosis
WHO	wrist-hand orthosis; World Health Organization
WHO-FIC	World Health Organization Family of International Classifications
wk	week
WNL	within normal limits
WP	whirlpool
WWP	warm whirlpool

Y

y.o. or yo	year old

SYMBOLS

about	~	less than, less than or equal to	<, ≤
after	$\overline{p}$	male	♂
ascend or increase	↑	micron	μ
assist (min, mod, max assist)	ⓐ, (a), or (A)	negative	(–) or —
at	@	not equal to, unequal	≠
before	$\overline{a}$	number of individuals assisting (one, two)	× 1, × 2
both or bilateral	bil., B, (B), or Ⓑ	parallel (as in parallel bars)	// (// bars)
degrees	°	per	/
degrees Celsius	°C	positive	(+) or +
degrees Fahrenheit	°F	possible, question, suggestive	?
dependent	(D) or dep.	pounds	# or lbs.
descend or decrease	↓	primary	1°
equal, equal to	(=)	right	Ⓡ, (R), or R
extension	/	sample mean	x
female	♀	secondary, secondary to	2°, 2° to
flexion	✓	times (as in 3 times per day)	× (eg, 3 × /day)
from	←	to	→
greater than, greater than or equal to	>, ≥	to and from	↔
hour, foot	'	up and down or ascend and descend	↑↓
inch, minute	"	with	$\overline{c}$
independent	(I) or Ⓘ	without	$\overline{s}$
left	Ⓛ, (L), or L		

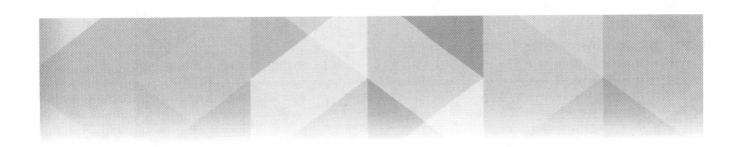

Index

Printed in the United States
by Baker & Taylor Publisher Services